Questions and Answers

in

SURGERY FOR STUDENTS

Questions and Answers
in
SURGERY FOR STUDENTS

M. J. Kelly
MChir FRCS MRCP
Senior Registrar in General Surgery,
Bristol Royal Infirmary

Gill Kelly
SRN
Ex-Senior General and Orthopaedic Ward Sister,
St. George's Hospital,
London

H. P. Henderson
FRCS
Senior Registrar, Plastic and Jaw Department,
Fulwood Hospital, Fulwood,
Sheffield

With a Foreword by
Professor R. Y. Calne
MS FRCS FRS

WRIGHT·PSG
Bristol   London   Boston
1981

M. J. and G. L. Kelly, Myrtle Cottage, Back Lane, Pill, Nr Bristol,
Avon.
H. P. Henderson, 12 Botanical Road, Sheffield S11 8RP.

Published by
John Wright & Sons Ltd., 42–44 Triangle West, Bristol BS8 1EX,
England
John Wright PSG Inc., 545 Great Road, Littleton, Massachusetts 01460,
U.S.A.

British Library Cataloguing in Publication Data

Kelly, M.J.
    Questions and answers in surgery for students.
    1. Pathology, Surgical - Problems, exercises, etc.
    I. Title   II. Kelly, Gill   III. Henderson, H.P.
    616′.00246171   RD57

ISBN 0 7236 0601 3

Printed in Great Britain by
Billing & Sons Limited, Guildford, London and Worcester

PREFACE

This book is intended to provide undergraduate medical students with a relatively painless method of revision for the surgery of their Final M.B. Examination. It also attempts to cross the enormous gulf that exists between the M.B. candidate and the competent house-surgeon. Senior clinicians tend to observe loftily that this kind of knowledge can only be learnt 'on the job' by apprenticeship, and consequently they feel absolved from teaching it. Certainly the standard short texts in surgery are strong on 'set-piece' disease entities, but startlingly light on decision making and patient management. Furthermore, to those of us who have been on the job after hours continually for the last ten years, their ideas are dated, and divorced from what we actually do.

Much of the houseman's expertise is acquired from his working with an experienced ward sister. The relationship is similar to that between a new subaltern and an experienced warrant officer, in that although the officer is technically the 'superior', he rarely over-rules the other, and then only at his peril. Consequently we feel that it is right and desirable that this book should be written by two surgical senior registrars and a ward sister. All of us know only too well the areas where medical students are uncertain,

and where newly qualified doctors are
frequently adrift. This book sets out at
least to confront you with some of the
problems in the way that they will present
to you when you have qualified.

Undergraduate medical teaching is
almost entirely the art of knowing what to
leave out, and how to simplify the remainder
without compromising the truth. We believe
that this can only be done if the teachers
are bold enough to define their objective.
In our view the aim of the undergraduate
curriculum should be to train a doctor to
the level of *Casualty Officer*, who has already
completed a medical and surgical house job.
This *Casualty Officer* should be able to
handle the seriously ill for about twenty
minutes until senior help arrives, and also
be competent at sorting out and pointing in
the right direction all the other patients.
Anything that is too detailed or specialised
for this *Casualty Officer* should be omitted
from his basic undergraduate curriculum. We
hope we have succeeded in applying this
stringent dictum to our book.

Although the accent and slant is
different, this present book forms a
companion volume to our *'Questions and Answers
in General Surgery'*, *Henderson and Kelly (1979)*
which is aimed at Final F.R.C.S. candidates.
Again we have used the format of questions and
short answers because we consider it to be so
much more flexible and useful to the reader
than M.C.Q.

We believe that the answers in this
book conform to the mainstream of good
current surgical practice. To this end we
have enlisted the help of the following
colleagues and friends at the senior

registrar/young consultant level from the
major specialist centres; any residual
shortcomings remain our own responsibility.

Anaesthetics, Fluid balance: J.H.W.Ballance FFARCS,
              Senior Anaesthetic Registrar,
              Bristol Royal Infirmary.
Arterial Surgery: R.J.Lusby FRCS FRACS,
              Research Fellow in Vascular
                Surgery,
              Bristol Royal Infirmary.
Bacteriology in Surgery: A.Davies MB BS,
              Senior Registrar in
                Microbiology,
              Southmead Hospital, Bristol.
Cardiothoracic Surgery: C.J.Hilton FRCS,
              Consultant Surgeon,
              Regional Cardiothoracic
                Centre, Newcastle.
Endocrine Surgery: M.H.Thompson MD FRCS,
              Lecturer,
              Bristol Royal Infirmary.
E.N.T. Surgery: P.D.Bull FRCS,
              Consultant E.N.T. Surgeon,
              Royal Hallamshire and
                Children's Hospitals,
                Sheffield.
General Surgery: W.E.G.Thomas MS FRCS,
              Senior Registrar,
              Bristol Royal Infirmary.
Gynaecology in Surgery: W.R.Tingey FRCS MRCOG,
              Senior Registrar,
              John Radcliffe Hospital, Oxford.
Haematology in Surgery: C.L.Rist MRCP MRCPath,
              Consultant Haematologist,
              Worthing.
Neurosurgery: D.T.Hope FRCS,
              Senior Neurosurgical Registrar,
              Frenchay Hospital, Bristol.
Ophthalmology: M.G.Kerr-Muir FRCS MRCP,
              Senior Registrar,
              Moorfields Eye Hospital, London.

Orthopaedic Surgery: C.J.Good FRCS,
                     Senior Registrar,
                     Rowley Bristow Hospital
                        Rotation,
                     Pyrford, Surrey.
Paediatric Surgery: A.E.MacKinnon FRCS,
                     Consultant Paediatric Surgeon,
                     Children's Hospital, Sheffield.
Rectal Surgery: M.R.Thompson MD FRCS,
                     Senior Registrar,
                     St. Mark's Hospital, London.
Transplantation Surgery: B.D.Pentlow MS FRCS,
                     Senior Lecturer,
                     Renal Unit,
                     Southmead Hospital, Bristol.
Urology: R.J.Morgan FRCS,
                     Senior Lecturer,
                     Urological Institute, London.
Everything: D.B.Shortland MB ChB,
                     House Surgeon,
                     Bristol Royal Infirmary.

Michael Kelly
Gill Kelly
Hugh Henderson

Acknowledgements

It is a pleasure for us to acknowledge
the continual help and encouragement we have
received from Dr John Gillman of Messrs John
Wright & Sons. We are very appreciative of
the unstinting assistance given to us by
Mrs Sheila Nichols, secretary in Bristol,
and Mrs Mary Walker in Doncaster. The final
version was typed 'for the camera' by
Mrs Mary Walker at Doncaster.

Table of Contents

Preface	iii
Foreword	vii
Acknowledgements	viii
How to use this Book	xi
General Surgery	1
Anaesthetics and Fluid Balance	79
Arterial Surgery	101
Bacteriology in Surgery	113
Cardiothoracic Surgery	127
Endocrine Surgery	147
E.N.T. Surgery	157
Gynaecology in Surgery	167
Haematology in Surgery	175
Miscellaneous and Nursing	181
Neurosurgery	195
Ophthalmological Surgery	209
Orthopaedic Surgery	225
Paediatric Surgery	249
Rectal Surgery	263
Transplantation Surgery	283
Urology	289
Index	313

FOREWORD

Professor Roy Yorke Calne MS FRCS FRS

In the last few years there have been several new publications designed to help the undergraduate and junior doctor understand and learn surgery. Some of these texts have departed from the traditional format indicating a dissatisfaction with the conventional didactic methods. I suspect that there is a place for both approaches, one providing the factual information and the other the more practical help for the man at the 'coal face' being confronted with new, perplexing and difficult clinical presentations.

The aim of this book, as stated in the preface, is for it to be of genuine practical help to senior students and house surgeons up to the level of Casualty Officer. Thus it can be used as a text to be read in the form of a quiz or alternatively, to be referred to via the index when a patient presents with certain symptoms and physical signs. The authors point out the analogy of the junior House Surgeon working with the Ward Sister as being similar to a subaltern working with a Warrant Officer. The Senior Registrar resembles a Company Commander and is likely to be of more practical help in patient management at a house officer level than the more experienced 'Commanding Officer', who seldom now has to set up a drip, pass a catheter or plan intravenous fluids and electrolytes.

The questions have been sensibly chosen; they are answered briefly and dogmatically. This is inevitable and must be accepted in a book of this length, there being no room for stating the evidence for an opinion and an analysis of conflicting ideas. I am sure that this book will be appreciated by senior students and surgical residents and the authors will feel that their efforts have not been wasted as they move from Company Commanders to Commanding Officers.

R. Y. Calne
Addenbrooke's Hospital
Cambridge

How to Use This Book

The questions are placed on the right hand page and the answers are to be found on the back of the same page immediately after turning over, making sustained 'cheating' less easy.

Following 'General Surgery', the sections on the various surgical specialties come in alphabetical order. Within each section an attempt has been made to group questions together in a logical sequence, although often this has been only partly possible.

An index has been provided at the end of the book to permit quick revision of topics that impinge on several sections in the book.

General Surgery

1. List a reasonable differential diagnosis for R.I.F. pain in a woman of 30 years who has never had previous surgery.

2. You admit a previously completely fit 21 year old lady with one day's history of central abdominal pain, moving to the right iliac fossa. She has vomited once, and there are no bowel, urinary or gynaecological symptoms. She has the signs of acute appendicitis. Ward testing of the urine is clear. What investigations should you do?

3. Patients with acute appendicitis usually do not have dysuria, but they often say that it 'hurts to pass water': explain.

1.   Acute appendicitis   ) often disting-
      Acute Meckel's diverticulitis) uishable only
      Acute ileo-caecal Crohn's   ) at operation

      Pelvic inflammatory disease,)
         salpingitis, tubo-ovarian)
         abscess   )
      Ruptured right ectopic tubal) gynae
         pregnancy   )
      Twisted right ovarian cyst   )
      Endometriosis   )
      Midcycle ovulatory pain   )

      Right ureteric colic)
      Cystitis   ) urology
      Pyelonephritis   )

      Gastroenteritis
      Rarities

2.   None.
      The chance of the chest x-ray being
         abnormal is very low.
      No finding on plain x-ray of the abdomen
         will stop you operating.
      The haemoglobin will be normal.
      No matter whether the w.b.c. is high,
         normal or low, you will operate.
      The likelihood of her urea being abnormal
         is remote.
      She needs analgesia and appendicectomy,
         but not tests.

3.   You may obtain a different answer depend-
         ing on how you phrase your question.
      Many appendicitis patients claim that it
         'hurts to pass water'. What they mean
         is that the act of micturition causes
         lower <u>abdominal</u> pain (due to local
         peritoneal irritation).
      Dysuria means true urethral pain ('as if
         the water burns').

4. Do you think vaginal examination is of
    much use in the diagnosis of the
    acute abdomen in young women?

5. Is a w.b.c. ever useful in assessing the
    acute abdomen?

6. What is mesenteric adenitis?

7. You admitted a 25 year old lady with
    "non-specific abdominal pain" and
    slight fever overnight. Today both
    have settled and you wish to send
    her home. Do you need to re-examine
    her?

4.   Yes, it is especially useful in this age
          group.
        A careful, gentle vaginal examination
          that takes up to 5 minutes will usually
          enable you to decide quite definitely
          whether there is, or is not, gynaeco-
          logical pathology. This may well alter
          the entire management of the case.
        If you are not sure, put the patient to
          bed, and repeat it after an hour or so.

5.   Yes, but not very often.
        a) If you wish to send the patient home
              from casualty, a high w.b.c. may
              stop you.
        b) In an abdomen with many previous scars,
              a high w.b.c. may suggest ischaemic
              bowel and hasten surgery.
        c) In the elderly with a possible mesen-
              teric infarction, high w.b.c. may
              hasten surgery.

6.   This is a common condition mimicking
          appendicitis, believed to be viral,
          characterised by abdominal pain and
          enlarged mesenteric nodes affecting
          children. It is usually only diagnosed
          at operation when the appendix is normal
          but the nearby nodes are enlarged. It
          is probably the abdominal manifestation
          of a mild generalised viral illness.

7.   Yes.
        Check that the fever has settled and the
          abdomen is soft.
        Repeat rectal examination (to exclude
          pelvic appendicitis).
        Repeat vaginal examination (sometimes you
          may now be able to feel the tender
          ovary which was the cause of her
          symptoms).
        Check that an M.S.U. has been sent.
        The patient may leave once she has eaten
          and kept the food down.

8. In preparing a patient for operation,
    what is a "through shave"? Is it
    necessary for an appendicectomy?

9. A twenty year old labourer underwent
    appendicectomy for an acutely inflamed,
    unperforated appendicitis, five days
    ago. His postoperative course has been
    uneventful and he is ready to go home.
    When do you advise him to return to
    work?

10. Name two signs of achalasia of the cardia
    seen on plain radiographs.

11. What does "primum non nocere" mean?

12. How would you treat a breast abscess?

8.   A "through shave" means removal of all
      the pubic hair, suprapubic, perineal
      and upper thigh. As any previous
      recipient will tell you, the regrowth
      of perineal hair is an uncomfortable,
      itchy business.
      A "through shave" is completely unnecess-
      ary for an appendicectomy. Only the
      "bush" needs removal down to the base
      of the penis/upper labia. One cannot
      extend the incision any lower, the
      symphysis pubis is in the way!

9.   In about 3-4/52.
      It is quite surprising how much the
      apparently trivial operation of appendi-
      cectomy prostrates the system even in
      the young and very fit. He will feel as
      if he has had a really bad attack of
      'flu, and will need this period to
      recuperate.
      Highly motivated individuals have gone
      back to work much earlier than this,
      but this is unusual.

10.   Absent stomach gas bubble.
      Fluid level seen behind the heart on a
      penetrated chest x-ray.

11.   "Above all do no harm".

12.   Incision and drainage under G.A.
      The early stage of diffuse cellulitis may
      be controlled by antibiotics
      (Flucloxacillin), but once pus is
      demonstrable by fluctuation, drainage
      becomes necessary.
      Lactation (if present) may be allowed to
      continue using a breast pump.
      In an older patient, any residual lump
      should be biopsied.

13.   Outline the classic features of a small
      fibroadenoma of the breast.

14.   Does the use of the contraceptive pill
      correlate with an increased incidence
      of breast cancer?

15.   Benign mammary dysplasia is very common.
      Give 3 synonyms for this condition.

16.   Outline the spectrum of the condition
      known as benign mammary dysplasia,
      and its management.

17.   How should you describe a lump?

13.   1-3 cm, painless, non-tender, bosselated,
        discrete lump in a young woman's
        breast.
      Mobile +++ (hence its description as a
        "breast mouse").
      Treatment is local excision which is easy.

14.   Numerous surveys all agree that the
        answer is "No".

15.   Fibroadenosis
      Chronic mastitis
      Fibrocystic breast disease

16.   a) Many women never have any trouble
         with their breasts.
      b) Many women have slight premenstrual
         breast discomfort only.
      c) Some women have (b) and once or twice
         in their lives have a benign discrete
         cyst or lump that requires aspiration
         or excision.
      d) Some women have marked cyclical breast
         pain and may need hormones or diuretics.
      e) A few women in (d) regularly make cysts
         and lumps and require careful super-
         vision by an experienced surgeon to
         strike a balance between excluding
         cancer and repeated excisions and
         biopsies of mastitic breast tissue.
      f) A tiny minority of (d) and (e) have
         such sustained trouble and form such
         diagnostic problems that eventually
         a mastectomy or subcutaneous mast-
         ectomy with breast reconstruction
         may be recommended.

17.   Site, shape, size, surface, sound (bruit).
      Consistency - solid, cystic, emptiable,
        pulsatile.
      Colour.
      Temperature, whether transilluminates.
      Attachments - superficial, deep.
      Regional lymph nodes.
      Distant effects.

18.   When you examine a lady of 28 years
with a breast lump, is it helpful
to know the date of her last period?

19.   How do you test for deep fixation of a
breast lump?

20.   What are the standard 4 criteria or
procedures that must be fulfilled
for aspiration of a cystic breast
lump to be safe?

18. Yes, often. The chances are that a 28
     year old woman will have either a
     fibroadenoma or benign mammary
     dysplasia.
     Cancer does occur in this age group but
     it is rare.
     If the lump is discrete and hypermobile -
     there is no difficulty. This is a
     fibroadenoma and should be excised.
     If the lump is less distinct, you have
     to decide whether it is a discrete
     lump meriting biopsy, or just the
     general induration of benign dysplasia.
     Pre-menstrually many women's breasts are
     quite lumpy so it is wise to re-examine
     them in mid-cycle, when such changes
     reach their minimum. If the induration
     persists mid-cycle then your patient
     needs surgical referral.

19. Ask the lady to place her hand on her
     hip.
     Grasp the lump and move it backwards and
     forwards, parallel to the fibres of
     pectoralis major, meanwhile ask her
     to press her hand hard on her hip and
     then release it. Look for tethering
     of the lump while she is pressing.
     Repeat the manoeuvre moving the lump in
     a plane at right angles to the first.
     To demonstrate deep fixation, you must
     elicit tethering in both planes.

20. 1. The fluid aspirated must not be
         blood stained.
     2. The lump must disappear completely
         afterwards.
     3. The fluid must be submitted to
         cytology.
     4. The breast must be re-examined in
         one month and the lump still be
         absent.
     When any of these 4 criteria are not
     fulfilled, excision biopsy is
     required.

21. Does an indrawn nipple matter?

22. Can anything be done about the cosmetic aspect of a nipple which has been chronically inverted since puberty?

23. What is the probable cause of bilateral nipple discharge of green toothpaste like material in a multiparous woman in her thirties?

24. Who should mark a breast lump prior to surgery? How should you make the mark?

25. Name some factors associated with an increased risk of breast cancer.

21. a) Sinister significance: long standing
         indrawn nipples are common and
         unimportant, but recent indrawing
         occurs with cancer and plasma cell
         mastitis. Biopsy is usually necess-
         ary.
     b) Function: suckling of an infant is
         difficult with an indrawn nipple.
         Breast abscesses may be commoner
         in these patients.

22. Using a periareolar incision the nipple
     can be detached from the breast ducts
     and stitched back nicely everted.
     These reconstructed nipples look
     good, but are often slightly numb and
     will not, of course, lactate.

23. Duct ectasia (plasma cell mastitis) - a
     benign condition which often causes
     severe distress.
     Treatment - excision of a plug containing
     the large ducts behind the nipple.

24. The surgeon performing excision should
     mark the lump himself. If he dele-
     gates it to the H.S., mark the skin
     with the patient lying in bed with
     her arm abducted, just as she will
     lie on the operating table.

25. Early menarche.
     Late first pregnancy.
     Positive family history of breast
     carcinoma.
     Past history of cancer in the other
     breast.
     Failure to breast feed (controversial).

26. How do you manage a woman of 38 who tells
     you she has eczema of the nipple?

27. How does intraduct papilloma of the
     breast present? Does it carry a
     good or bad prognosis?

28. When are mammograms indicated?

26.   Be very suspicious that this is really
       Paget's Disease of the nipple - the
       local change caused by an underlying
       breast cancer.
      Examine her completely naked for any
       evidence of other patches of eczema,
       and especially for any lump under
       the nipple of the affected breast.
      Arrange a mammogram and chest x-ray.
      Provided there is no palpable lump
       prescribe a strong steroid ointment,
       and allow a maximum of 3 weeks for
       it to heal the 'eczema' (which it
       will do if it is true eczema).
      If unimproved after 3 weeks, refer for
       urgent biopsy. In Paget's Disease
       the histology is diagnostic.

27.   Discharge of blood from a single nipple
       duct.
      Treated by microdochectomy - a careful
       radial dissection of the duct and
       its segment of gland, leaving the
       rest of the breast.
      These papillomata usually present early
       (because the blood is frightening)
       and if they have not breached the
       basement membrane the prognosis is
       good.

28.   Mammography is a controversial subject;
       it is probably of little value once
       a decision has been taken to remove
       a lump.
      a) Well women screening: $>$ 35 years. (In
          younger women, films are more diffi-
          cult to interpret).
      b) Breast diseases:
          Recurrent breast lumps, especially
          after multiple local excisions.
          Lumpy breasts which are difficult
          to assess.
          Large breasts which are difficult
          to palpate.
          Persistently painful breasts to
          exclude localised pathology.

29. What does mastectomy offer a woman with
     breast cancer?

30. Radical mastectomy for Stage I and II
     carcinoma of the breast as an
     initial procedure is seldom per-
     formed nowadays. What alternative
     methods of surgical treatment are
     considered acceptable (in the belief
     that survival and dissemination rates
     are no worse)?

31. In which group of breast cancer patients
     has adjuvant endocrine or chemo-
     therapy been shown to reduce recur-
     rence and probably improve survival
     if given at the time of surgery?

32. As there are minimal differences in
     long-term survival between the
     differing types of breast cancer
     operation, why is lumpectomy not
     the obvious solution?

29.   Mastectomy (simple, Patey, radical)
       ± radiotherapy is to control the
       local disease and stop chest wall
       recurrence. Long term survival
       depends on whether unremoved
       seedlings were present at the time
       of surgery and tumour/host response.

30.   a) Wide local excision and radiotherapy
          in Stage I disease (Guy's trial).
       b) Simple mastectomy and watching policy
          in Stage I and II (King's/Cambridge
          trial).
       c) Simple mastectomy supplemented by
          radiotherapy only when there is
          proven involvement of pectoral or
          lower axillary nodes (Cardiff trial).
       Reference: *Forrest A.P.M. Conservative*
       management of breast cancer: A review
       of British controlled trials. Annals of
       R.C.S. Engl.1980 62 *41-43.*

31.   Premenopausal patients.
       Reference: *Hayward J.L. Radical breast*
       surgery, 1980. Annals of R.C.S. Engl.
       62 *43-45.*

32.   Lumpectomy is an amazingly difficult
       policy to operate. The operation is
       associated with an increased incidence
       of local recurrence.
       The patients must be closely followed up
       and this generates an enormous O.P.D.
       load.
       Follow up examination is incredibly
       difficult because one is left trying
       to decide whether the misshapen remains
       of the breast contain recurrent tumour
       or not. This leads to multiple x-rays
       and biopsies which further compound the
       problems.
       With mastectomy ± DXR the local problem
       is over and finished with for patient
       and doctor alike.

33.   Compare the prognostic significance
       of recurrence-free intervals for
       breast and colonic cancer after
       treatment.

34.   Distinguish between the words
       'incidence' and 'prevalence'.

35.   It can be helpful to distinguish two
       types of patient with bedsores.
       Those at high risk of recurrence,
       and those at low risk.
       Give examples of each, and briefly
       indicate the difference in manage-
       ment.

33.   Although it is an over-simplification,
      and not absolutely true, a patient
      surviving 5 years, recurrence free
      after 'complete' excision of a
      colonic cancer, is probably cured.
      Breast cancer continues to have a
      recurrence rate for at least 15
      years. It is not infrequent for a
      mastectomy patient to live 10 years
      recurrence free, only to develop
      liver secondaries, deteriorate and
      die within 6 months.
      The reasons for this disparity are
      unknown.

34.   Incidence: number of cases occurring
                 during a specific period
                 in a specified population.

      Prevalence: all cases detected at a
                  particular time in a given
                  population.

35.   High risk of recurrence: Paraplegics,
      immobile senile geriatric patients
      and incontinents.

      Low risk: Fit young patients with
      bedsores after prolonged periods
      of unconsciousness, head injury,
      overdoses etc.

      The first group must either be trained
      to look after themselves more care-
      fully, or else nursed more intensively.
      They tend to require vitamins, iron
      injections and transfusions to aid
      healing.
      The second group is unlikely to suffer
      the same problem again, and merely
      requires rapid treatment of the sore.
      Surgery may be helpful and secure an
      early cure.

36.   What is the single main cause of bed
      sores? How do you treat them?

37.   In a patient with marked ascites,
      what is the easiest way to confirm
      that its origin is malignant?

38.   What do you understand by the term
      'occult carcinoma'?

39.   Can gall stone colic be felt in the
      left hypochondrium?

36. Virtually all experienced ward sisters
     of all ages will tell you that bed
     sores are due to inadequate nursing.
     Many features predispose (cachexia,
     immobility, incontinence etc.) but
     sustained, careful nursing can cope
     with all of these. A nurse away at
     a meeting cannot prevent bedsores.
     Management:
     a) Careful nursing; 2 hrly 'turning';
         reducing pressure by the use of
         special beds such as ripple beds,
         waterbeds or low-loss air beds.
     b) Culture swabs and treatment of
         Strep. and *Staph.* only. Isolation
         of patients with other bacteria.
     c) Attention to general nutrition.
     d) Sometimes plastic surgery recon-
         struction may be necessary.

37. Aspirate 20 cc and send for cytology.
     The cytologist will usually be able
         to suggest a site of origin e.g.
         ovary.
     Whether you then 'hunt the primary'
         depends on many factors; not least
         the philosophy of your consultant.

38. A carcinoma whose secondary or systemic
         effects present before the primary
         tumour is identifiable, e.g. vertebral
         collapse due to secondaries in a lady
         who later develops an identifiable
         breast carcinoma.

39. Yes, but it is uncommon. The gall
         bladder and bile ducts develop as
         outpouchings of the foregut and
         therefore have bilateral visceral
         innervation.

40.   A plain x-ray of the abdomen taken for
      another reason shows an asymptomatic
      opaque gall stone. What should you
      do?

41.   Oral cholecystogram and intravenous
      cholangiogram show different
      aspects of biliary function.
      Outline their uses.

42.   What dose of Papaveretum (Omnopon)
      would you prescribe for a patient
      with severe pain from cholecystitis?

40. The management depends on an estimate
     of the relative risks of chole-
     cystectomy versus the morbidity and
     mortality of possible cholecystitis
     and jaundice.
     a) old person, generally unfit for
         elective surgery - no treatment.
     b) remainder - oral cholecystogram
                     $\pm$ intravenous cholan-
                     giogram.
     Functioning gall bladder + stones - open
         to discussion.
     Non-functioning gall bladder + stones -
         probably needs operation.
     Stone in common bile duct - needs
         operation.

41. Oral cholecystogram outlines a func-
         tioning gall bladder well, but only
         gives hazy detail of the CBD.
         Hypersensitivity risk low.
     IVC outlines the CBD, but frequently
         gives only hazy detail of the GB.
         Hypersensitivity risk higher,
         anaphylaxis even - but still low.
     Oral cholecystogram is the standard
         OPD method of diagnosing gall
         stones, whereas IVC is the usual
         in-patient investigation for a
         patient with acute cholecystitis
         (cystic duct already blocked).
     Many patients require both.
     Neither can be used in a deeply
         jaundiced patient.

42. Papaveretum is not used as a first
         choice in this condition because
         one of its actions is to increase
         smooth muscle spasm. Thus Pethidine
         is usually prescribed (50-100 mg
         i.m. 4 hourly).

43. Are there any indications for urgent
     surgery in patients with gall
     stones?

44. Suggest how the likelihood of a gall
     stone being present in the CBD may
     have logistic importance for the
     H.S. in arranging an operating list.

45. When should you remove a surgical
     drain?

43.   Yes, but they are somewhat infrequent.
       Absolute - perforated gall bladder.
                - increasing obstructive
                  jaundice due to stone(s)
                  in CBD.
                - gall stone ileus.
       Relative - severe cholangitis, unrespon-
                  sive to antibiotics.
                - increasing right upper quadrant
                  peritonism, despite conserva-
                  tive management.
       Controversial - a policy of urgent
                  cholecystectomy in patients
                  with cholecystitis.
                  (This is logistically, techni-
                  cally and practically far
                  more difficult to execute
                  than to propose!)

44.   This is important information for those
           planning the firm's operating list.
       CBD exploration alters the category
           from intermediate to major and means
           that the operation needs to be done
           by a consultant or experienced (S)Reg.
           and adds at least $\frac{3}{4}$ hr. to the
           procedure. The list will need to be
           organised to permit this senior
           supervision.

45.   The standard examination room answer is
           "when it stops draining"; but in
           practical terms add the words "when
           the surgeon who inserted it directs".
       Remember that drains are inserted for
           different reasons (e.g. to drain
           haematoma, drain bile, form a track)
           and that consequently the reasoning
           behind time of removal also differs.
       Drain removal is an irrevocable step
           and should first be sanctioned by the
           operator.

46.   How would you remove a T-tube from
      the common bile duct post-
      operatively?

47.   Define "hernia".

48.   Which anatomical landmark helps you
      to distinguish between inguinal
      and femoral hernia?

49.   Differentiate irreducible, obstructed,
      or strangulated hernia.

46.   Check i) the date of operation: it is
               unusual to remove a T-tube
               before the 8-10th post-
               operative day because the track
               may not have adequately sealed
               off from the peritoneal cavity.
          ii) normal postoperative T-tube
               cholangiogram x-ray.
        iii) that your seniors have indeed
               authorised removal.

Obtain an assistant who can get help
    if there are difficulties.
Insert a butterfly needle and give a
    small dose of pethidine i.v.
Cut the stitch retaining the T-tube.
Give the tube a firm hard pull. It
    should slide out with minimal
    resistance. If it does not, have
    another 2 tries, but if you are
    pulling like mad, and the patient
    is writhing round the bed, something
    is wrong, and you need senior help!

47.   A hernia is an abnormal bulging of a
        viscus or tissue into another across
        a tissue plane.

48.   The pubic tubercle. The neck of an
        inguinal hernia lies above and
        medial to the pubic tubercle,
        whereas that of a femoral hernia
        lies below and lateral (because
        the fascial layers cause the femoral
        hernia to turn round on itself as it
        enlarges).

49.   Irreducible: not reducible, contents
                   viable, often contains
                   only omentum.
    Obstructed: bowel obstructed, but viable,
                 hernia usually irreducible.
    Strangulated: obstructed + impaired
                  blood supply (i.e. ischaemic
                  contents).

50. How does the treatment of inguinal
     hernia vary with the age of the
     patient?

51. What is the usual underlying cause
     of an incisional hernia?

52. Which of the commoner abdominal hernias
     are particularly prone to strangu-
     lation? Is there some common
     denominator among them?

53. Which 3 things may easily be confused
     with a femoral hernia?

54. How would you treat a true umbilical
     hernia in an infant of 6 months?

50.   Infants, children: All congenital,
           indirect hernias. Remove sac only.
       Young adults: Usually indirect, strong
           muscles. Remove sac, minimal
           reinforcement of muscles.
       30-60 years: Usually indirect, remove
           sac, also need repair of canal.
       60+years: Some indirect as above.
                 Some direct - wide sac, push
                 back only. Need repair of
                 canal $\pm$ orchidectomy (especially
                 if recurrent).

51.   Infection or haematoma in the wound.
       This causes a partial disruption of the
           deep layers which does not proceed
           as far as a true burst abdomen but
           ends up as an incisional hernia
           which later enlarges.

52.   1) Femoral
       2) Paraumbilical
       3) Indirect inguinal
       4) Epigastric
       5) Incisional
       They all have a narrow neck to the
           hernial sac.

53.   Inguinal hernia (note relation to pubic
           tubercle).
       Saphena-varix (surprisingly easy to
           confuse: standing, a tap impulse
           passes up LSV to the lump).
       Lymph node (may be impossible to
           differentiate).

54.   Provided it is not gross and is easily
           reducible (the usual case), manage
           conservatively. By one year most
           will have disappeared. Those
           remaining by about 18 months - 2
           years should be repaired electively -
           an easy operation.

55.   What is a Richter's type hernia?
      In which variety of hernia is
      it commoner? Why is it import-
      ant?

56.   You have a patient as a 'long case'
      in your examination who confi-
      dently tells you that, as well as
      thirty other problems, he has a
      hiatus hernia. What symptoms
      should you enquire about in case
      the examiner asks you?

57.   The management of hiatus hernia
      represents one of the unsolved
      problems of surgery. Why is this?

55.   Only a portion (e.g. half) of the
      circumference of the bowel wall
      is caught and strangulated by the
      neck of the hernia.
      It is commoner in femoral (11% of
      strangulated ones) than inguinal
      (3% of strangulated ones).
      Gangrene of the strangulated portion
      of bowel wall may occur in the
      absence of intestinal obstruction.
      The dead wall then tears and the
      bowel falls back, leading to gross
      peritonitis.

56.   Heart burn.
      Regurgitation, especially on bending
      forward.
      Dysphagia.
      Bleeding.
      Vomiting.
      Dyspepsia.

57.   There are 3 facets:
      a) Symptoms - reflux, pain etc.
      b) Radiological signs - reflux, actual
         hiatus hernia.
      c) Endoscopic signs - oesophageal
         redness.
      The problem is that a, b and c do not
      correlate well. Thus, not only do
      many patients have b and c, but not
      a, and some the reverse; but even
      in those with underlying symptomatic
      proven hiatus hernia, surgical
      correction is often impermanent and
      the degree of subjective improvement
      is often unrelated to any objective
      changes in b and c.

58. Are any of the following types of
     hernia suitable for management
     by a truss, and if so, why?
     Indirect inguinal
     Direct inguinal
     Femoral
     Paraumbilical
     Ventral incisional

59. Define a hamartoma.

60. Classify haemorrhage.

61. What is the primary treatment of
     haemorrhage?

62. Your team decides to operate on a 65
     year old patient referred from the
     physicians with melaena who has
     received 12 units of blood over
     the last 3 days. Do you need to do
     any coagulation tests?

58. A truss may be a very useful 'second
     best' to surgery where either the
     patient is too unfit for operation
     or repair is unlikely to work
     (e.g. chronically infected recurrent
     ventral hernia).
     However, a truss can only exert simple
     inwards pressure at right angles to
     the pressure plate, thus it is suit-
     able for direct straight bulges, but
     not for obliquely sliding ones.
     Truss suitable: direct inguinal, some
                     indirect
                     ventral incisional
     Truss unsuitable: many indirect inguinal
                     (oblique bulge)
                     femoral (oblique bulge
                     + narrow neck)
                     paraumbilical (narrow
                     neck + sl oblique)

59. A hamartoma is a non-neoplastic
     malformation characterised by an
     abnormal mixture of tissues
     indigenous to the part with an
     excess of one or more of these,
     e.g. bronchial hamartoma, keloid.

60. Primary   Arterial   External
     Reactionary   Venous   Internal
     Secondary   Capillary

61. PRESSURE. Only if adequately applied
     local pressure fails to control
     the bleeding need you have recourse
     to more sophisticated treatment such
     as pressure-point control, tourni-
     quets etc.

62. Probably yes - the patient has received
     what amounts to an exchange trans-
     fusion.
     Simple platelet screen + prothrombin
     time are probably adequate.

63.   How would you control severe bleeding
       from a thigh wound?

64.   You have admitted a 60 year old man
       after a marked haematemesis.
       After initial resuscitation
       endoscopy shows an active D.U.
       with blood clot over it. His
       condition is now stable: P.80,
       B.P. 150/95. What instructions
       do you give the night nurses?

63. a) Pressure: cover the wound with
        bandages, handkerchief etc. and
        press. If the blood soaks
        through, do not remove the cloth,
        but apply another on top.
     b) If local pressure fails, apply a
        tight tourniquet proximally,
        making a written note of the time,
        provided it is removed within one
        hour it is absolutely safe, and
        has saved many lives.
     Prohibitions on its use stem from the
        particular conditions pertaining
        to World War I warfare!

64. You must be specific in your require-
        ments and give precise figures.
     Observations: ½ hrly P., hourly B.P.,
        4 hrly temperature and respiration,
        if patient has naso-gastric tube
        2 hrly aspiration. Stool chart.
     Tell them that you wish to be woken
        and told if:
     1) Further large haematemesis or
        melaena, or patient feels very
        faint.
     2) Pulse > 105 for 2 consecutive
        readings.
     3) B.P. < 110 systolic for 2 con-
        secutive readings
        (N.B. (2) & (3) These figures will
        vary from patient to patient, but
        you must set actual limits.)
     4) Anything else that worries the
        nurses.
     Make it quite plain that you would
        far rather be woken up in error
        than left to sleep while the patient's
        condition deteriorates.

65. Give an outline summary of the house surgeon's contribution to the management of a major gastro-intestinal bleed in Casualty.

65. 1) If you know in advance that the
        patient is coming, tell your
        registrar and warn the blood
        transfusion service.
     2) On seeing the patient assess the
        gravity of the hypovolaemia:
        (i)   patient conscious P.$<$120,
              B.P.$>$95$\Rightarrow$you can manage on
              your own for a bit.
        (ii) patient conscious P. 120-140
              B.P. 70-95$\Rightarrow$you need two
              people.
        (iii) patient unconscious P$>$140
              B.P.$<$60$\rightarrow$you need all the
              senior people available.
     3) Instruct the casualty staff to
        ensure that the ambulance men remain
        until you have questioned them.
     4) Set up a large saline drip, 14 gauge
        or better.
     5) Through the same needle take at
        least 30 ml blood for tests.
        If you cannot obtain this quantity,
        take it by femoral vein puncture.
     6) Do haemoglobin, U. & E., cross match.
     7) Cross match at least 3 units of blood
        for all haematemeses. Alter this
        amount when the haemoglobin result
        becomes available.
     8) If B.P.$<$80, commence a plasma
        expander i.v. (e.g. PPF, haemacel.).
     9) If you have not already called your
        registrar, do so now.
    10) Interview ambulance crew and see
        what blood, if any, was passed in
        the ambulance.
    11) Inform the duty anaesthetist.
    12) By now you have to have senior help
        present. If you cannot find the
        appropriate person, keep going up
        the ladder until you get somebody.
        In this situation if no-one else is
        to be found, your consultant will
        always come himself.

66.   You are told to check that a medical
      patient with a haematemesis has
      "sufficient" blood cross-matched.
      How do you calculate this figure?

67.   Your team has successfully operated
      on a lady with severe bleeding
      from a D.U. It is now the third
      post-operative day, and she is
      doing well. Do you need to warn
      her about anything regarding her
      first few bowel actions?

66.   Hb. values do not fall immediately
       with major bleeds, but they do
       drop quite markedly within 24
       hours and are usually some guide.
1) Look through the notes/G.P.'s
   letters to see if there was a
   previous Hb result from the past.
   i.e. is there also chronic anaemia?
2) Estimate roughly how much blood
   has been lost (difficult).
3) Note current Hb.
   1 unit of transfused blood raises
   Hb. by approximately 1 g%. You
   also need 3 units of blood in the
   'fridge as a reserve against the
   next bleed and to cover any
   operation.
   e.g. 3 large vomits of blood +
        1 melaena Hb 9 g%
        You need: 12 - 9 = 3 units to
        restore Hb. to low normal (12g%)
        + 3 units operative reserve for
        next bleed = 6 units of blood
        total.

67.   Yes.
       Your patient has had an emergency
          operation to stop melaena.
       The intestines remain filled with
          blood, so the first bowel move-
          ments will still be very offen-
          sive melaena.
       If you forget to warn your patient,
          she will naturally assume that
          the bleeding continues and the
          operation has failed!
       Meantime you must check the Hb on
          alternate days to make sure it
          is steady and that she is really
          not bleeding!

68. When you have a patient in the I.T.U.,
     are there any specific logistic
     problems you need to bear in mind
     when arranging your day's activities
     and organising his care?

69. What is Troisier's sign?

70. What are the main varieties of
     malignant tumour affecting the
     liver?

71. List the commoner causes of a local-
     ised hepatic swelling.

68.   The problem with I.T.U. patients is
        liaison and communication. Find
        out the policy in your I.T.U.
        regarding who looks after which
        aspects of patient care. Also
        discover your own team's attitude
        to that policy!
        Advice:
        a) Go to the I.T.U. before anywhere
           else first thing in the morning.
        b) Each time you visit, write in the
           notes.
        c) Make sure the staff know which
           member of your firm is available.
        d) Refer policy decisions to your
           seniors with despatch.

69.   The involvement of the left supra-
        clavicular lymph nodes by meta-
        static tumour (these are also
        called Virchow's nodes). The
        primary is often carcinoma of the
        bronchus or carcinoma of the stomach.

70.   Secondaries (the vast majority of liver
           tumours).
        Hepatoma.
        Cholangiocarcinoma (carcinoma of the
           bile ducts).
        Lymphoma.

71.   2° carcinoma (these make up at least
           90%).
        Hepatoma.
        Riedel's lobe (an anatomical variant).
        Hydatid cyst.
        Amoebic abscess.

72.   Is there any point in putting the
      patient to the discomfort and
      slight risk needed to obtain a
      tissue diagnosis of multiple
      hepatic secondaries when the site
      of the primary neoplasm is uncertain?

73.   What does the abbreviation S.O.S. on
      a prescription chart mean?

74.   A cystic hygroma is a rare lymph-
      angiomatous malformation. Where
      would you expect to find one and
      which physical sign does it
      demonstrate par excellence?

75.   What is likely to be the cause of a
      midline cystic swelling in the neck
      that moves on swallowing and on
      protrusion of the tongue?

76.   What does acholuric jaundice mean?

72.   Yes.
      a) A tissue diagnosis makes it much
         easier to give a prognosis and
         frequently makes effective handling
         of patient and family far easier.
      b) A few histology reports carry a
         better prognosis:
         i)   Lymphoma - may respond to
              treatment
         ii) Carcinoid - may go on for years
              with established liver second-
              aries.
      c) The diagnosis may be wrong. The
         "multiple hepatic secondaries" may
         occasionally be cysts or other
         pathology.

73.   Latin: "si opus sit" = if the situation
      should arise. It is similar to
      p.r.n. = "pro re nata" - if the
      thing occurs.

74.   In either supraclavicular triangle of
      the neck - in a child.
      It is brilliantly and unmistakably
      transilluminant.

75.   A thyroglossal cyst.

76.   Jaundice without bile in the urine
      (a - chol - uric)
       no bile   urine
      It is characteristic of haemolytic
      anaemia where there is an excess
      of circulating unconjugated
      bilirubin.

77.   Distinguish between prehepatic,
      hepatic and post-hepatic
      jaundice. Does this distinc-
      tion matter?

78.   List some of the commoner causes of
      post-operative jaundice.

79.   What is Courvoisier's 'law' in
      obstructive jaundice?

77.   Prehepatic - excess unconjugated
                   bilirubin (fat soluble).
                   urine bile negative,
                   urobilinogen +
                   SAAT = Alk. Pa = normal.
       Hepatic   - excess conjugated and
                   unconjugated bilirubin
                   SAAT ++; Alk. Pa +
       Post-hepatic - excess conjugated (water
                   soluble) bilirubin
                   SAAT normal, Alk. Pa +++
                   bile in urine, no uro-
                   bilinogen.
       The distinction is important.
       Prehepatic and hepatic jaundice are
          treated medically.
       Post-hepatic = obstructive jaundice,
          usually requires surgical correction.
       (N.B. drug induced cholestatic jaundice
          has many of the features of obstruc-
          tion.)

78.   Biliary/hepatic surgery: retained stones,
          oedema/spasm of the ampulla of Vater.
          Operative damage to the common bile
          duct.
       Absorption of sequestered blood; e.g. after
          successful repair of leaking aneurysm.
       Anaesthetic: halothane.
       Blood transfusion problems and, much
          later, serum hepatitis.
       Infection: when gross with haemolysis.
                  Hepatitis (if the indication
                  for surgery was erroneous).

79.   It is important to get the negatives
          correct.
       "In obstructive jaundice, if the gall
          bladder is palpable, the obstruction
          is unlikely to be due to gall stones".
       The theory is: gall stones ⟶ episodes
                      of cholecystitis
                      ⟶ small thick walled
                      impalpable gall bladder.
                      Ca. pancreas ⟶ continu-
                      ous, unremitting
                      obstruction ⟶ enlarged
                      palpable gall bladder.

80. How is malignant obstruction of the
     CBD treated?

81. Which solid tumours can now be treated
     principally with chemotherapy with
     a reasonable hope of extended
     remission or even 'cure'?

82. Give an outline list of the causes of
     a post-operative pyrexia in an
     adult.

83. Describe the presentation of a patient
     with a mesenteric infarction.

80.   Ca. head of pancreas: 90% cases of
      malignancy obstructing CBD.
      R$_x$ - usually by-pass procedures -
      GB to jejunum etc.
      Ca. ampulla of Vater: Rare, diagnosed
      at endoscopy and biopsy.
      R$_x$ - Whipples pancreaticoduoden-
      ectomy - a huge operation with a
      good ultimate prognosis in this
      subgroup.
      Ca. common bile duct: Rare, radical
      surgery of some form may be curative.
      The tumour is slow growing even if
      it cannot be removed completely.

81.   Chorioncarcinoma.
      Disseminated Hodgkins.
      Burkitt's lymphoma.
      Mycosis fungoides.

82.   Infection - operation site: haematoma,
                      anastomotic leak etc.
                   wound
                   chest
                   pelvic, subphrenic abscess
                   urine - catheter, instru-
                      mentation
                   I.V. infusion
      DVT
      Blood - haematoma, transfusion reaction
      Drug reaction

83.   The patient is usually old.
      Acute, severe abdominal pain, vomiting,
      diarrhoea ± blood. There is often a
      history of cardiac disease. Tempera-
      ture may be normal or low; hypo-
      tensive or shocked. Abdominal
      distension ++, abdominal tenderness
      but little guarding. Sometimes a
      source for the emboli is apparent
      (e.g. A.F., S.B.E., recent myocardial
      infarct) but more often none is
      identified. The predominant impres-
      sion is of severe pain with prostra-
      tion in an old patient with relatively
      less dramatic abdominal physical signs,
      but with a markedly raised W.B.C.

84.   Have you ever seen post-operative acute
      dilatation of the stomach? If not,
      why not? Do you think you would
      remember it if you had? Describe it.

85.   Give an outline classification of the
      causes of intestinal obstruction.

86.   Name the 3 commonest causes of intestinal
      obstruction.

87.   What differentiates paralytic ileus from
      mechanical intestinal obstruction?

84.   Probably not, and you will certainly
      remember it if you have!
      It occurs two to three days post-
      operatively and the stomach fills
      with 4-6 litres of foul dark fluid,
      some of which may be vomited. It
      presents as abdominal distension
      with profound collapse and hypo-
      tension, which can lead to
      inhalation and death.
      The selective routine use of naso-
      gastric tubes in major abdominal
      surgery has almost (but not com-
      pletely) abolished this dread
      complication.
      Remember that if your patient collapses
      unexpectedly with some abdominal
      catastrophe, pass a nasogastric tube.
      If he has gastric dilatation you will
      aspirate 4-5 litres and cure him.

85.   a) Dynamic: compression from outside
            bowel wall - hernia, adhesions,
            volvulus, intussusception etc.;
            compression from the bowel wall
            itself - carcinoma, stricture etc.;
            blockage of the bowel lumen -
            impacted stone, polyp, foreign
            body etc.
      b) Adynamic: paralytic ileus,
            mesenteric vascular occlusion.

86.   Carcinoma, hernia, adhesions.

87.   A patient with paralytic ileus has
      effortless vomiting of large
      amounts, no colic, and absent
      bowel sounds.

88. What is a paralytic ileus? Outline
     the stages of resolution.

89. List 4 classical symptoms of complete
     mechanical obstruction.

90. Do you think strong analgesics
     (e.g. Pethidine, Papaveretum)
     should ever by given to patients
     with bowel obstruction?

88.   Ileus is a form of adynamic intestinal
      obstruction. The intestines stop
      absorbing and peristalsing and
      slowly distend with chyme. 'Full
      blown' ileus is marked by absolute
      constipation, painless silent
      abdominal distension, effortless
      vomiting of large quantities of
      brown discoloured fluid.
      Resolution is marked by the reversal
      of these features.
      NGT aspirates decrease, become clear
      and cease.
      Oral fluids are retained without
      nausea.
      Abdominal distension disappears and
      bowel sounds reappear.
      Flatus, diarrhoea and ultimately normal
      stools are passed.

89.   Abdominal colic.
      Vomiting.
      Abdominal distension.
      Absolute constipation.

90.   Yes, but with caution because they
      will mask the signs of strangu-
      lation which often form the major
      indication to abandon conservative
      management and operate.
      a) As premedication once a decision
         has been taken to operate.
      b) One or two doses to tide the patient
         over the night once it has been
         decided to postpone the decision to
         operate from say 11.00 p.m. to
         8.00 a.m.
      c) Only with senior sanction, in cases
         of recurrent intestinal obstruction
         due to adhesions from multiple
         operations.
      (What you must not do, and it is a very
      easy mistake, is to write up
      Pethidine 4 hourly, and forget the
      problem!)

91.   How long should intestinal obstruction
      without an obvious cause be treated
      conservatively?

92.   Are the fluid and electrolyte changes
      of small bowel obstruction reason-
      ably predictable and, if so, what
      are they?

93.   What are the classical signs of a
      malignant parotid tumour?

94.   Which important structure is at risk
      in parotidectomy?

95.   Outline the presentation of congenital
      pyloric stenosis. Do such infants
      usually require referral to a
      Regional Centre?

96.   With what aphorism did John Hunter
      describe the stomach?

91. Complete obstruction
     + peritonism - immediate operation.
     - peritonism - small bowel - delay
                              up to 12 hours
                    large bowel - delay
                              up to 24/36 hours
     Incomplete obstruction
     + peritonism - immediate operation
     - peritonism - small bowel - delay
                              12 - 24 hours
                    large bowel - delay
                              up to several days

92. Yes, to a large extent they are the
     changes associated with prolonged
     vomiting, i.e.
     a) Fluid loss $\longrightarrow$ hypovolaemia, oliguria.
     b) K^+ loss in the vomit $\rightarrow$ hypokalaemia.
     c) HCl loss in the vomit $\rightarrow$ metabolic
        alkalosis.
     However, their extent varies from case
        to case, consequently measurements
        need to be made each time.

93. A hard, irregular swelling with skin,
        VII nerve and lymph node involve-
        ment.

94. The facial nerve. Damage causes
        weakness or paralysis of the
        muscles of facial expression, the
        mouth and blinking.

95. Congenital pyloric stenosis presents
        at 4-6 weeks of life with increasing
        projectile vomiting (usually) in
        male first born children.   Diagnosis
        depends on feeling the 'duodenal
        olive' during a test feed. Operative
        management lies well within the
        capabilities of most district
        general hospitals.

96. A gland with a cavity.

97.   List the commoner methods of
      presentation of a gastric
      carcinoma.

98.   In which country is there a signifi-
      cant incidence of superficial
      gastric cancer, in which resect-
      ion produces far better results
      than in most other gastric cancers?

99.   In general, gastric cancer has a very
      poor 5 year survival rate.   Are
      there any gastric neoplasms which
      have a favourable prognosis?

100. What is the action of Cimetidine
      (Tagamet)?

101. Why do some duodenal ulcers perforate
      and others bleed?

97. 1) General malaise with weight loss
        and mild iron-deficiency anaemia.
     2) Epigastric pain, worse with eating.
     3) Non-specific dyspepsia.
     4) Epigastric mass which may be the
        primary lesion, or liver second-
        aries or both.
     5) Haematemesis or melaena.
     6) Vomiting.

98. Japan.

99. Yes, but they are rare.
     Benign lesions: leiomyoma, neuroma,
        lipoma etc.
     Malignant lesions: lymphoma, superficial
        spreading mucosal gastric carcinoma -
        diagnosed by endoscopic biopsy.

100. Cimetidine is a histamine-H_2 receptor
        antagonist, and it inhibits resting
        and stimulated gastric acid
        secretion.

101. It is due to their anatomical position.
     Consider 2 ulcers each penetrating a
        centimetre. The anteriorly placed
        one will erode the full thickness
        of the duodenal wall and perforate,
        whereas the posterior one will
        erode the retroperitoneum and into
        the gastroduodenal artery.

102.   What principles govern the operative
        treatment of a perforated D.U.:
        and how may an H.S.'s clerking be
        important in determining it?

103.   Should one persevere with conservative
        treatment of a gastric ulcer for a
        similar period of time to that which
        one allows a duodenal ulcer?

102.   The primary purpose of the operation
       is to close the hole and save the
       patient's life. The quickest,
       easiest and safest way to do this
       is by simple oversewing of the
       ulcer with an omental flap.
       However, if this is all you do,
       more than 60% of chronic ulcers
       will later recur.
     The second purpose of the operation
       is to use this opportunity to
       perform whatever definitive
       operation the patient's ulcer
       diathesis demands, ignoring the
       acute event. Thus the H.S.'s
       clerking noting chronic ulcer
       symptoms, may indicate a need for
       some acid reducing procedure rather
       than simple oversewing, and this is
       usually the case.
     The actual operation done is determined
       by the fitness of the patient and
       the experience of the surgeon.

103.   No.
     5-10% of gastric ulcers believed on
       endoscopy, biopsy, barium, to be
       benign, are in fact malignant.
       Whereas, for practical purposes,
       duodenal ulcers are never malig-
       nant. Thus it is reasonable to
       spend many months trying to coax
       a D.U. into healing realising the
       risks are of bleeding, perforation
       and narrowing, not malignancy.
       Contrariwise, if a G.U. has not
       healed after 4-6 weeks conservative
       treatment, excision should be
       considered as the only certain way
       of excluding malignancy.

104.   What are the indications for surgery
        for a duodenal ulcer?

105.   What are the generally accepted
        indications for emergency surgery
        in a patient admitted with a
        bleeding D.U?

106.   A middle aged man tells you he has had a
        'gastric operation' but he now com-
        plains that soon after eating he feels
        distended and often hears abdominal
        'rumbles'. If he carries on eating
        his discomfort worsens and occasionally
        he feels sick and vomits. Usually he
        feels tired and faint and wants to lie
        down. He often perspires, pants and
        suffers diarrhoea but within an hour or
        so he feels better.
        What does this history suggest?

104.   a) Absolute - perforation.
                     - repeated bleeding that
                       continues.
        b) Relative - duodenal/pyloric stenosis.
                     - chronic pain leading to a
                       disruption of life style
                       with failure of medical
                       treatment.

105.   a) Absolute - severe exsanguinating
                       bleeding with which
                       transfusion cannot
                       keep abreast.
                     - continued marked bleeding
                       that needs transfusion
                       and fails to stop.
        b) Relative - signs of a large re-bleed
                       in hospital (this means
                       that after admission and
                       resuscitation, there is
                       another fresh haematemesis
                       or melaena).
                     - Continued slow bleeding
                       evinced by a falling Hb.
                       requiring repeated trans-
                       fusion.
                     - Transfusion of 'a lot' of
                       blood over a short period
                       e.g. more than 8 units in
                       2 days.
        Old people stand the stress of massive
        preoperative blood loss and trans-
        fusion less well than younger and so,
        paradoxically, one's operative
        threshold is lower in these elderly
        patients.

106.   The early dumping syndrome. It is
        probably caused by over rapid
        emptying of the stomach.

107.   How would you carry out a provocation
       test for 'dumping'?

108.   Outline your approach to the problem
       of the patient with recurrent pain
       after ulcer surgery.

109.   Post-gastrectomy symptoms are divided
       into 2 types, a) post-cibal;
       b) metabolic. What are the
       important features of each type?

107.   After starving the patient from
       midnight, the patient is given
       150 ml of 50% glucose for break-
       fast. The patient is observed
       and asked to report if his
       symptoms are mimicked by this
       fluid meal. The haematocrit should
       be measured every 10 minutes during this
       period; a fall in plasma volume
       greater than 14% is highly suggestive
       of dumping.

108.   Start afresh with a repeat full history
       and careful examination. Try to
       discover whether the patient's
       symptoms are the same as those
       preceding the ulcer operation or
       different. Establish whether there
       was a pain-free period after the
       operation.
   Then:
     1) consider whether the original
        diagnosis of peptic ulcer was
        wrong, and investigate other
        possibilities, e.g. gall stones.
     2) discover whether there is
        objective evidence of a recurrent
        peptic ulcer - endoscopy, barium
        meal.
     3) see whether there is an identi-
        fiable cause (e.g. acid studies
        incomplete vagotomy, Zollinger-
        Ellison).

109.   a) Post-cibal - early dumping.
                       late hypoglycaemia.
                       bilious vomiting.
       b) Metabolic - small stomach, reduced
                       intake, weight loss.
                       diarrhoea/steatorrhoea/
                       malabsorption.
                       Fe deficiency) most
                         anaemia   ) patients
                       B_{12} deficiency) need
                         anaemia   ) supple-
                       Ca deficiency) ments

110.　You are called to casualty to see a
known ulcer patient who is
prostrated with sudden onset of
severe generalised abdominal pain.
What is the likely diagnosis? How
should you pursue it?

111.　What are the commoner causes of
recurrent peptic ulceration
following surgery?

112.　Describe primary and secondary
Raynaud's phenomena.

110.   Perforated D.U.
        1) Set up a drip.
        2) Give a small amount of intravenous
           analgesia (say Pethidine 5-15 mg
           i.v.).
        3) Pass a nasogastric tube and empty
           the stomach to reduce further
           leakage.
        4) Arrange erect and supine abdominal
           x-rays to seek free gas.

111.   a) Either the first operation was
           inadequate in design or execution.
           e.g. incomplete vagotomy (assess
           by insulin stimulated acidity test);
           partial gastrectomy may fail to
           remove the antrum or enough of the
           parietal cell mass.
        b) Or it was the wrong operation,
           e.g. vagotomy inappropriate in the
           Zollinger-Ellison syndrome or
           G-cell hyperplasia; gastroenterostomy
           alone is probably the wrong operation
           for uncomplicated D.U.

112.   Episodes of pallor, followed by cyanosis
        and painful redness of the extremities
        induced by exposure to cold or emotion
        (due to vascular spasm).
        Primary (Raynaud's Disease): females,
           intermittent, bilateral, no gangrene,
           no underlying disease. Rarely bad
           enough to merit surgery.
        Secondary: often unilateral, sclero-
           derma, 'collagen diseases', cervical
           rib, vibrating tool injury.
           Often do need surgery.

113.   What is the purpose of debridement
       of wounds?

114.   Injuries ascribable to explosions
       are usually divided into 2 groups,
       direct and indirect. Explain.

115.   List the common causes of free gas
       under the diaphragm.

116.   What is the commonest abnormality
       picked up by a full Family
       Planning Centre well-women
       screening programme?

113.   To remove all devitalised tissue and
       foreign bodies (which tend to
       promote infection and impede wound
       healing). Muscle and skin that
       fail to bleed when the tissue
       perfusion of the patient is other-
       wise normal should be excised.
       Dirt becomes fixed to the tissues
       within a few hours, and irrigation
       is then insufficient to clean the
       wound. Dirt left in the skin may
       not prevent healing but will leave
       ugly tattoos.

114.   Direct or primary blast injury is due
       to the direct impact on the tissues
       of variations in atmospheric
       pressure from the explosion. These
       injuries involve the lungs and ears
       mostly.
       Indirect injury can be sub-divided
       into those
       a) from missiles (secondary blast
          injury).
       b) whole body displacement (e.g. the
          body tossed into the air; tertiary
          blast injury).
       c) miscellaneous effects (quaternary
          blast injury, e.g. burns,
          asphyxiation etc.).

115.   1) Perforated D.U.
       2) Perforated G.U.
       3) Perforated diverticulitis.
       4) Perforated carcinoma of the colon.
       5) Recent laparotomy/laparoscopy.

116.   Breast lumps. About four times more
       breast lumps are found than cervi-
       cal smear abnormalities. Thus
       breast palpation is an important
       part of the screening.

117.   Does acute pancreatitis give a 'full
       blown' generalised peritonitis,
       or is the syndrome less dramatic
       and consequently easy to stop?

118.   How do you manage a case of severe
       acute pancreatitis?

119.   What is a collar stud abscess?

117.   Acute pancreatitis can produce a <u>very</u>
       variable picture from a localised
       to a fulminant generalised periton-
       itis.
       Established acute pancreatitis results
       in the release of activated pan-
       creatic enzymes both into the
       retroperitoneum and onto the anterior
       surface of the gland, the lesser sac.
       Thus there is a marked chemical
       peritonitis which is often indis-
       tinguishable from a perforated
       peptic ulcer. Diagnosis depends
       on the finding of a preoperative
       serum amylase $\geqslant$1000 S units.

118.   This condition is usually diagnosed
       before any operation has taken
       place and is managed conservatively.
       "Drip and suck" replacement of fluid
       and electrolytes (to treat ileus)
       with monitoring of U. & E., Ca^{++},
       blood gases and urine output.
       Transfusion to replace blood lost
       retroperitoneally.
       Analgesia+ antispasmodics (e.g. Pethidine
       +Atropine).
       Glucagon.   )
       Protamine (Trasylol)) controversial
       Antibiotics   )
       When the patient goes home:-
       a) No alcohol for at least one year.
       b) Look for gall stones and treat
       where appropriate.
       Acute pancreatitis is a serious
       condition with a mortality rate
       of over 10%.

119.   A subcutaneous infection with a deep
       subfascial loculus (forming the
       base of the 'collar stud'). It
       can occur anywhere and is typical
       of Tb. neck lymph node infection.

120.   Describe how you would remove a lump
       from the scalp diagnosed as a
       'sebaceous cyst' by one of your
       predecessors.

121.   Is the commercially available mixture
       of lignocaine-adrenaline useful?
       Are there any circumstances where
       it might be dangerous?

122.   In an examination you are shown a
       'short case' of an elderly man
       with a lesion on his forehead
       which is 1 cm. diameter, has a
       raised rolled edge, ulcerated
       centre with crusting. What is
       the likely diagnosis and differ-
       ential diagnosis?

120.   Satisfy yourself that the lump has no
        deep attachment, and if in any
        doubt, take a check skull x-ray
        first.
        Shave around the area.
        Briefly wash your hands, and infiltrate
        the skin locally with lignocaine-
        adrenaline mixture.
        Now scrub up fully, and arrange your
        drapes.
        Incise an ellipse of skin to include
        the punctum, and try to remove the
        cyst intact by scissor dissection.
        If you do burst it, carefully remove
        all the retained cyst wall by artery
        forceps traction.
        Tie off any obvious bleeding vessels
        and press in the wound with a swab
        soaked in some more of your
        anaesthetic mixture.
        Insert a few sutures, with a drain if
        it was very large.
        No dressing is usually needed.

121.   Yes, very useful. The adrenaline is
        added in a very low dose 1/100,000
        suitable for stopping local arteriolar
        bleeding, e.g. face, mouth, perineum.
        Dangers:
        1) it should not be used in patients
        known to have cardiac problems.
        2) check drug medications. Adrenaline
        is very dangerous with many drugs
        especially MAO inhibitors.
        3) care must be taken not to inject
        large volumes intravenously.
        4) it must never be used where end
        artery spasm may lead to gangrene
        e.g. digits or penis.

122.   Basal cell carcinoma (rodent ulcer).
        Differential diagnosis: squamous cell
        carcinoma, intra-epithelial carcinoma.
        amelanotic malignant melanoma,
        keratoacanthoma.

123.   How may a B.C.C. be treated?

124.   Why is it important to establish
        quickly whether or not a patient
        with haematemesis may have bleeding
        oesophageal varices? What princi-
        ples then govern management?

125.   Classify shock.

123. a) deep curettage with histology
         (dermatologist)
      b) local irradiation (radiotherapist)
      c) simple excision and suture (general
         surgeon)
      d) excision with flaps or grafting
         (plastic surgeon)
      If you are not sure which is appropriate,
      ask the dermatologist's opinion first.

124. Because bleeding oesophageal varices
         may cause fatal exsanguination
         within a matter of a quarter hour.
      Management:
      1) Put up 2 large effective drips.
      2) Cross match at least 10 units of
         blood.
      3) Try to establish whether varices
         are known to be present from the
         history, examination, old notes.
      4) Early gentle endoscopy by <u>an expert</u>
         to see whether it is the varices
         that are bleeding or other pathology,
         e.g. D.U.
      5) Early correction of clotting defects.
      6) Early referral to regional unit.
         + Sengstaken tube, vasopressin etc.
         The mortality for a large bleed is
         over 50%

125. a) Hypovolaemic(blood, plasma or water
         loss).
      b) Cardiogenic (myocardial infarct,
         arrhythmia, tamponade, late hypo-
         volaemia, pulmonary embolus, general
         anaesthesia).
      c) Septic.
      d) Peripheral pooling (relatively rare
         but possible, especially in spinal
         shock or spinal anaesthesia).

126.   What are the main features in common, and distinguish the main differences between hypovolaemic, cardiogenic and septic shock?

127.   What is the cause and natural history of peri-anal warts? What are the alternative treatments?

128.   List the types of operation for reduction of morbid obesity.

126.   Features in common:
        B.P., urine flow, pH all fall.
        Pulse, blood lactate rise (pulse
            may occasionally fall).
        Differences:
        Cardiogenic & hypovolaemic:
            cyanosed/cold/sweaty/vasoconstricted.
        Septic shock:
            bounding pulse/warm/flushed.
        CVP tends to fall in hypovolaemic and
            septic shock, but rises in cardio-
            genic shock.
        A-V oxygen difference rises in hypo-
            volaemic and cardiogenic shock, but
            may fall in septic shock. P_aO_2 falls
            in hypovolaemic and cardio-
            genic shock, but may remain normal
            till late in septic shock.

127.   Cause: viral infection of peri-anal
            or anal skin.
        Natural history: most warts persist
            untreated, causing perineal
            discomfort, irritation and
            occasional bleeding. A few regress
            spontaneously. Malignant change
            can occur but is rare.

        a) Excision of wart bearing skin with
           some form of closure.
        b) Careful excision of each wart
           raised on a bleb of injected saline.
        c) Diathermy.
        d) Cryotherapy.
        e) Application of podophyllin solution.

128.   Reduction of intake of food: jaw
            wiring (It sounds harsh and is
            not without risk, but it is
            effective in the short term).
        Reduction of absorptive surface -
            by-pass procedures, small bowel
            resections, gastric reduction
            operations.

        Lipectomies are seldom used in the
            treatment of obesity, only in the
            cosmetic removal of redundant skin
            folds when massive weight loss has
            been achieved.

129.   What are the daily carbohydrate,
       fat and protein requirements
       of the universal 70 kg man at
       rest?

130.   How do you grade muscle power?

131.   How would you manage a drunken patient
       with a small puncture wound in the
       right upper quadrant of the abdomen?

132.   Why may a patient with a ruptured
       spleen complain of shoulder
       tip pain, especially if the
       bed is tipped a little head
       down?

129.   Approximately:
        CHO 300 g   fat 60 g   protein 50 g
        Multiply by:
          x 4   x 9   x 4   to obtain
        calories.

130.   0 - total paralysis
        1 - barely detectable contraction
        2 - insufficient to overcome gravity
        3 - just sufficient to overcome
              gravity
        4 - stronger than 3 but less than
              full power
        5 - normal

131.   The stage is set for you to perpetrate
          the classic error of taking this
          lightly.
        You cannot tell from the size of a
          stab wound how long the blade was.
        Never probe these in casualty, and
          never, never stitch and send home.
        Refer to the duty surgeon who will
          admit the patient overnight.
        He will explore the wound and proceed
          to laparotomy if the clinical signs
          and investigations (including
          peritoneal lavage and abdominal
          x-rays) indicate this.

132.   A ruptured spleen bleeds intra-
          peritoneally. Such blood runs
          back along the under surface of
          the diaphragm. The suprascapular
          nerves share common roots with the
          phrenic (C 3,4 5) which is both
          motor and sensory. Consequently,
          irritation of the diaphragm may
          cause pain referred to the shoulder
          tip.
        Similarly a girl with a ruptured
          ectopic pregnancy may also have
          shoulder pain.

133.   How far up your list of priorities
        do abdominal and/or rib x-rays
        come in your immediate management
        of a patient with a suspected
        ruptured spleen?

134.   How long after operation should skin
        sutures be removed? Will this
        period vary for different
        operation sites?

133.   Pretty low down.
       Your patient needs:
       1) A good i.v. line.
       2) Cross matched blood.
       3) Resuscitation.
       4) Clinical assessment by senior
          people.
       5) Possible peritoneal lavage.
       6) Chest x-ray to exclude pneumothorax.

       Abdominal x-rays will only show the odd
          rib fracture and unless there is an
          associated pneumothorax, this
          information will not influence the
          immediate management.

134.   The purpose of skin sutures is to
          appose the wound edges accurately
          while healing commences. Each
          stitch hole itself forms a small
          scar which becomes more prominent
          the longer the stitch is left in
          situ. Removal is therefore a
          compromise between this scar and
          the risk of the wound falling apart.
       Factors to consider are the load-stress
          on the wound, blood supply of the
          part, adverse healing factors
          (e.g. diabetes) and cosmetic aspects.
       Face and neck 2-3/7
       Breast, superficial wounds)
       Skin-crease wounds   ) 5-6/7
          (e.g. appendicectomy)   )
       Laparotomy, thoracotomy wounds 10-12/7
       Diabetic amputation stumps 3/52

       N.B. An intradermal or subcuticular
          suture may be left in permanently
          if of absorbable material (i.e. Dexon),
          or for several weeks if of non-
          absorbable material (i.e. Prolene or
          Nylon).

135.   State the important principles
       governing the immediate manage-
       ment of a patient with a 25%
       burn.

135.   25% skin surface burn constitutes
        a major burn.
        Immediate resuscitation -
          i.v. line
          replacement with fluids: plasma,
            blood, saline, dextrose.
        Low dose i.v. analgesia (e.g. Pethidine
          10-20 mg ½ hrly) till conditions
          stable. Except during dressings,
          pain is usually not gross.
        Measure urine output, osmolality.
        Baseline tests: Hb, P.C.V., urea,
          electrolytes, weight.
        Cross match blood.
        Assessment of size of burn (rule of 9's).
        Calculate daily i.v. fluid requirement
          (usually large, e.g. 4-6 litres on
          the first day in an adult).*
        Measure P_aO_2, P_aCO_2 if inhalation burn
          likely to be present.
        Discussion with and transfer to a
          regional burns unit.
        Mortality of a 25% full thickness burn
          is 25% approximately in the elderly.

        *The Muir and Barclay formula gives an
          approximate guide to the volume of
          fluid that should be given in each
          of the first three four-hour periods,
          and the subsequent two six-hour
          periods following a burn.

$$\frac{\text{Volume}}{\text{per period}} = \frac{\text{weight of Pt. (Kg) x \% Area of Burn}}{2}$$

Anaesthetics and Fluid Balance

136. You will find that sometimes the anaesthetist does not see the patient until she reaches the anaesthetic room, and you are required to prescribe pre-medication. State the standard regimen, and indicate a minimal acceptable anaesthetic assessment.

137. If tomorrow's operating list contains a patient for a bilateral varicose veins operation, is there any special detail the anaesthetist will wish to know?

138. When you send a patient with acute intestinal obstruction to theatre for an operation, what will the anaesthetist expect you to have done to facilitate induction of anaesthesia?

136.   For the average fit woman: Papaveretum
       (Omnopon) 15 mg i.m. and Hyoscine
       (Scopolamine) 0.3 mg i.m. 1 hour
       before operation.
       History: Chest, heart.
                Previous operations and
                anaesthetics.
                Drugs taken, especially
                anti-depressants, anti-
                hypertensives, contraceptive
                pill.
                (patients should continue <u>all</u>
                doses of antihypertensive
                treatment, especially beta-
                blockers, including 0600 dose
                on morning of operation, even
                when "starved").
                Allergies. Family allergies.
                Dentures.
       Examination: chest and heart.
       Results: Hb, urea, chest x-ray, E.C.G.
       <u>N.B.</u> if you find adverse features you
            must insist that an anaesthetist
            assesses the patient pre-operatively.
            In cases of difficulty, the duty
            anaesthetic S.H.O. will suffice.

137.   Whether the surgeon intends also to
       tie the short saphenous veins.
       These lie in the popliteal fossa.
       The patient will have to be turned
       prone and will require endotracheal
       intubation.

138.   Passed a nasogastric tube and instituted
       aspiration. Inhalation of vomit is
       a real hazard in these cases, and
       an early attempt to empty the
       stomach is most helpful.

139.   What is a Biers Block?
        What type of anaesthetic is it?
        Does it have any special advantages
            in the reduction and manipulation
            of wrist fractures?

140.   What do you ask a patient before
            injecting him with a local
            anaesthetic agent?

141.   What are the important complications
            of the use of injected local
            anaesthetic?

139.   Biers Block is an intravenous
          regional analgesic block.
       After venepuncture circulation to
          the limb is occluded by cuff
          and an intravenous infusion of
          local anaesthetic is given into
          the isolated limb.
       The main advantage is that as this
          is not a <u>general</u> anaesthetic
          there is no need for any delay
          after food or drink, and the
          patient may be sent home more or
          less immediately afterwards.

140.   Always ask whether he has had local
          anaesthetic before and if he had
          a reaction to it. A small but
          significant number of patients
          are allergic to local anaesthetics.

141.   A) <u>Local complications</u>:
       1. Local oedema, inflammation, abscess
             formation, necrosis, gangrene,
             either from neglect of sterile
             precautions, use of vasoconstric-
             tive agents when contra-indicated,
             or toxic contamination of the
             anaesthetic agent.
       2. Trauma of injection - haematoma,
             nerve injury, pneumothorax etc.
       3. Mistaken solutions - accidental
             mis-identification of solutions/
             syringes.

       B) <u>General complications</u>:
       1. Allergic reactions.
       2. Toxic reactions from excessive
             dosage CNS - tremors, convulsions,
             respiratory depression: CVS
             myocardial depression, hypo-
             tension.
       3. Psychogenic - injections are often
             initially painful and some
             patients faint.

142. How may the fact that a patient has
      sickle cell disease affect the
      administration of any general
      anaesthetic?

143. Setting up intravenous drips can be
      difficult for the inexperienced.
      What simple manoeuvres do you
      know to help you find a vein and
      insert the cannula in difficult
      cases?

142.   Sickle cell disease is relatively common among persons of West Indian descent, and all such patients should have a screening test (it only takes ¼ hour), especially before emergency surgery.

In sickle cell disease the haemoglobin crystallises into a "sickle" under conditions of hypoxia. Consequently hypoxic episodes must be strenuously avoided, including tourniquets. In practice, sickle cell +ve means that the anaesthetic should be given by a senior clinician and not by a junior trainee even when the surgical condition is relatively trivial.

143.   We have all set up drips 'in a flash' on our own when rushed, but once you have discovered that the venepuncture is difficult, you must slow down.

You need a quiet patient, a decent light, an assistant and plenty of time.

Use a small bleb of local anaesthetic placed away from the vein so that the patient does not flinch at your attempts.

Ensure venous filling by using a sphygmomanometer inflated to a sub-diastolic pressure, and not a simple tourniquet.

Warming the limb in a bowl of hot water may occasionally be useful.

Insert the cannula through the skin in one movement, and into the vein as a second discrete one. Do this reasonably decisively, otherwise you will tend merely to invaginate the vein wall.

Know when to give up! If you do not succeed in three attempts, go and have a cup of coffee. If your next attempt fails, summon assistance.

144.   Assuming he is reasonably competent,
        why may the H.S. have difficulty
        in setting up an i.v. infusion?

145.   Are there any groups of patients
        where a careful H.S. should be
        reluctant to attempt to set up
        an i.v. drip without authoris-
        ation by his seniors?

144.   Inexperience: the commonest reason.
        One has to set up many hundreds
        of drips before becoming really
        proficient.
        Local factors: obese patients.
                        previous attempts
                         obscuring the field.
                        "small veins".
                        unco-operative patient.
                        thick or thin walled
                         veins.
        General features: vasoconstriction due
                         to hypovolaemia,
                         fever, cold etc.
                        oedema.
        (The duty anaesthetist S.H.O. can often
         be coaxed into giving assistance to
         a H.S.)

145.   Yes.
        When he really thinks he is going to
            fail (all the reasons cited above).
        Babies and children under 5 years -
            these drips are very precious and
            are usually set up by senior
            clinicians.
        Arterial surgery patients when there
            is any question of an arm vein
            being used as a vein graft to an
            artery.
        Patients for very major surgery where
            the elbow veins should be preserved
            for possible long lines.
        Burns - a cut-down is often needed.
        Private patients - these patients'
            contract is with the consultant and
            the careful H.S. is wiser not to
            perform any manoeuvre without his
            approval.

146. In order to understand fluid balance,
      you must appreciate normality.
      In the standard 70 kg man how is the
      sum made up of fluid input(s)
      versus fluid output(s)?
      Express these in two columns of figures
      which must tally.

147. What are the metabolic consequences
      of anuria?

148. Which groups of people in hospital
      are probably the best suited to
      setting up really difficult i.v.
      drips?

146.   Input per day

Oral fluid   2,000 ml
Water of metabolism   500 ml
  ($CHO \rightarrow CO_2 + H_2O$)
                                    _____
                                    2,500 ml

Output per day

Urine   1,500 ml
Faeces   400 ml
Insensible losses   600 ml
  (lung vapour,
   sweat)
                                    _____
                                    2,500 ml

147.   1) Over-hydration (water is not being
          excreted in the urine).
       2) Metabolic acidosis (fixed acids
          such as sulphates, phosphates
          derived from protein breakdown are
          no longer being excreted).
       3) Uraemia - urea is a CNS depressant
          (and also itself an osmotic
          diuretic).
       4) Hyperkalaemia - causes cardiac
          irritability and predisposes to VF.
       5) Sodium retention - difficult to
                             manage
                           - often compounded
                             by attempts to
                             correct the
                             acidosis with
                             $NaHCO_3$ which
                             contains much Na^+.

148.   Adults: the anaesthetists (especially
               those in ITU). Setting up
               i.v. drips under adverse
               conditions is a major part of
               their skill.
       Babies: either the paediatrician or
               paediatric anaesthetist.

149. Distinguish between oliguria and
      anuria.
      Does post-operative oliguria matter?
      How would you manage it?

149.   Oliguria =   500 ml in 24 hours.
       Anuria   = no urine at all.

Most post-operative patients have a
    degree of oliguria (due to being
    starved pre-op. and ADH secretion).
    In low risk patients one is prepared
    to wait 24 hours after operation for
    spontaneous voiding.
Patients at high risk of renal damage
    (e.g., after big operations, hypo-
    tensive episodes) need more active
    management. The big risk is of
    over-hydration. Severe acidosis
    takes some days to develop.
Bladder palpable suprapubically →
    coax into voiding, or catheterise.
Bladder not palpable - give small dose
    of Frusemide 20 mg i.v. or i.m.
        → bladder palpable as above
        → bladder still impalpable -
    catheterise.
After catheterisation make sure the
    hydration is adequate.
A CVP line is often needed.
Measure urine output hourly. If
    hourly total is < 20 ml for two
    readings there is oliguria
Give a provocation test of either
    drug diuretic (Frusemide) i.v. or
    osmotic diuretic (Mannitol) or
    fluid load (500 ml   normal saline
    in ½ hour).
If you cannot produce a diuresis after
    trying all of these, your patient
    has established oliguria. Seek
    senior help and limit fluids to
    output + 500 ml, keeping CVP
    normal

150.   Outline a standard intravenous fluid
       regime for the first 24 hours after
       a trouble-free partial gastrectomy
       that did not require blood trans-
       fusion.

151.   Are there any metabolic consequences
       to the presence of a biliary T-tube?
       What action ,if any, should you take?

150.   3,000 mls. of fluid - 2,000 mls is the
                            bare minimum.
                          - 1,000 ml extra is
                            added to counteract
                            pre-operative
                            starvation and
                            losses from the
                            swabs, evaporation
                            etc.

       50 mmol Na^+
       30 - 50 mmol K^+

       1,000 ml Dextrose saline + 10 mmol
         KCl 8 Hourly
                        or
       1,000 ml 5% Dextrose + 10 mmol KCl)
         in 8 hours   )
         500 ml normal saline + 5 mmol KCl)
         in 4 hours   )
         500 ml 5% Dextrose + 5 mmol KCl)
         in 4 hours   )
       1,000 ml 5% Dextrose + 10 mmol KCl)
         in 8 hours   )

       Each regime gives the same quantities
         of water, K^+, Na^+, but the former
         is far less wasteful of nursing
         time.

151.   Bile is rich in potassium.
       Action: 1) Remember to include the
                  volume of bile lost in
                  your daily fluid balance
                  requirements.
               2) Measure plasma (K^+) every
                  third day until T-tube is
                  removed.
               3) Once the track is sealing
                  off, elevate the bag to
                  waist height, and use the
                  tube as an overflow sump.
                  This will reduce the quantity
                  of bile lost.
               4) Long term biliary T-tube
                  patients probably need
                  potassium supplements.

152.   What time of day are urinary catheters
        traditionally removed and why?

153,   Is bedside measurement of urinary
        specific gravity much use to
        the surgeon?

154.   How do you interpret these post-
        operative figures in a 20 year
        old patient explored for a
        ruptured spleen and found to
        have merely a minor mesenteric
        bruise - Hb 11g, Urea 3, Na 119,
        K 3.1, HCO_3 20?
        What intravenous regime would you
        advise?

152. First thing in the morning (e.g.
     6.00 a.m.) and never at week-
     ends.
     Reason: if the patient voids
             spontaneously there is
             no problem.
             if retention recurs, this
             will be by the afternoon
             when staff are available
             to assess it, and perhaps
             recatheterise.
             Catheter removals at other
             times cause severe logistic
             upsets!

153. Yes, provided you do not ask too
     much of this simple test.
     The test is immediate and repeatable.
     The results are unreliable if there
        is too little urine, or if it is
        blood stained.
     a) Post-op. oliguria - high SG suggests
        fluid depletion.
     b) Post-op. diuresis after a period of
        hypotension -
        SG   1016 - high - suggests active
        diuresis eliminating metabolites
        R$_x$ continue fluids.
        SG   1005 - very low - suggests
        diuresis eliminating water
        R$_x$ reduce fluids.
        SG 1010 - suggests lack of renal
        concentration   diuresis of
        resolving tubular damage.
        R$_x$ high fluid/high urine output
        (diuretic phase of acute renal
        failure).

154. Overhydration.
     The patient was probably regarded as
        having intraperitoneal bleeding
        and given 1 - 2 litres of clear
        fluid before it became apparent
        that the injury was trivial.
     Intravenous regime: limit fluid (e.g.
        1,500 ml D-Saline + 25 mmol
        KCl/24 hours) and allow the
        patient's metabolism to sort
        itself out.

155.   Does the usual management of hypo-
       kalaemia differ from that of
       hyponatraemia?

156.   What two things may the finding of
       a low 'plasma sodium estimation'
       indicate?

157.   How much Mannitol should you give
       in order to provide a challenge
       and induce an osmotic diuresis?

158.   What is the hepato-renal syndrome?
       Is it important in surgery?
       What standard steps are taken to
       prevent it?

155.　Yes. Remember that these figures
　　　are concentrations and not
　　　absolute values.
　　　Low K$^+$ concentration is usually due
　　　to loss of K$^+$and requires K$^+$
　　　supplements.
　　　Low Na$^+$ concentration is usually due
　　　to excess water.
　　　R$_x$ - fluid restriction (hypertonic
　　　saline is a dangerous fluid. It
　　　tends to push elderly patients
　　　into heart failure and needs to
　　　be used only very rarely).

156.　Correctly this is a plasma sodium
　　　concentration. It means there is
　　　less Na per ml of plasma.
　　　Causes - a) Reduced Na in normal
　　　　　　　　plasma volume.
　　　　　　　b) Normal Na in increased
　　　　　　　　plasma volume.
　　　　　　　c) Combinations of a) and b).

157.　20 g. as a bolus over 20 minutes
　　　i.e. 200 ml of 10%) trickling it in
　　　　　100 ml of 20%) over an hour is
　　　　　　　　　　　　　not nearly as
　　　　　　　　　　　　　effective as
　　　　　　　　　　　　　running it in as
　　　　　　　　　　　　　a bolus.

158.　Hepato-renal syndrome is the associ-
　　　ation of severe renal failure with
　　　liver failure i.e. jaundice.
　　　Acute oliguria and uraemia is the
　　　major cause of death in jaundiced
　　　patients undergoing large operations.
　　　Prevention is by:-
　　　a) Ensuring adequate hydration with
　　　no episode of hypotension.
　　　b) Catheter to ensure complete measure-
　　　ment of urinary output.
　　　c) Mannitol induced osmotic diuresis
　　　before, during and after operation
　　　to retain an adequate urinary output
　　　($>$30 ml/ hr.) and thus 'protect'
　　　the kidneys.
　　　Use of this regime has virtually elimin-
　　　ated the post-op. hepato-renal syndrome.

159.   Define 'shock' in a single sentence.

160.   A cut-down on the long saphenous
       vein at the ankle is an amazingly
       easy, life saving little operation,
       provided you know where to look
       for the vein.   Where does it lie?

161.   The subclavian vein is frequently
       used as the site for an intra-
       venous 'long line'.
       List the complications which may
       arise from this procedure.
       Do they outweigh the benefit?

159.   Shock is a state produced by sudden
        reduced perfusion of vital organs.

160.   One fingers breadth <u>anterior</u> to the
        <u>medial</u> malleolus, accompanied by
        the saphenous nerve (sensory).
        There are no arteries here.
        (We have all seen frenzied
        ignorant people 'ring barking'
        the lateral calf looking for
        this vein!)
   N.B. Do not use a leg vein in prefer-
        ence to an arm vein without a good
        reason. Cannulated leg veins
        thrombose readily and are thought
        to predispose to D.V.T.

161.   a) Pneumothorax.
        b) Hydropneumothorax (with the
              contents of the drip pouring
              into the thoracic cavity or
              mediastinum).
        c) Local haematoma including arterial
              bleeding.
        d) Phrenic nerve damage.
        f) Subclavian vein thrombosis (rare).

        Once a subclavian line has been
           successfully set up it is both
           convenient for the patient (both
           arms are free), short in length
           and trouble free. Complications,
           as listed above, may be very
           severe and even, on occasional,
           life threatening.
        In general terms, the decision to
           use the subclavian site should
           be taken by senior personnel and
           usually only in the confidence
           that the other hemithorax is
           completely intact.

162. When calculating the optimal
      parenteral nutrition of
      seriously ill patients, what
      separate items should be
      considered?

162.   Total fluid volume requirements
        (taking account of renal
        function).
        Total calorie requirements.
        Minimal protein or nitrogen
        requirements.
        Phosphate requirements.
        Electrolyte requirements especially
        Na^+, K^+, Ca^{++}, and Mg^{++}, (taking
        account of previous serum levels
        and urinary output).
        Acid Base balance.
        Vitamins, iron, antibiotics and
        other drugs.

Arterial Surgery

163.   When the main artery to the leg
       becomes blocked, and the leg
       is not viable through acute
       ischaemia, how long does it
       take before the ischaemia
       becomes irreversible?

164.   Assessment of an acutely ischaemic
       leg in an old person is often
       made difficult by the knowledge
       that the peripheral pulses were
       absent before the current acute
       event. Which two physical signs
       are the best indicators that the
       leg is still viable?

165.   If you had severe intermittent
       claudication of one leg, would
       you prefer your femoral pulse
       to be present or absent on that
       side?

166.   In the case of suspected arterial
       embolism to a limb, what are
       the danger signs of severe
       ischaemia which indicate immedi-
       ate action to attempt to save
       some degree of function?

163.   About 6 hours. In other words,
        there are about 6 hours from
        the onset of severe symptoms
        during which emergency surgery
        may save the leg.

164.   Skin sensation present.
        Voluntary movement of the muscles
        present.

165.   Absent.
        If all the pulses in the leg,
        including the groin, are absent,
        you have an occlusion of the
        iliac vessels or aorta. Because
        your leg is viable, only giving
        exercise pain, the distal
        collateral circulation is good;
        consequently an arteriogram
        would probably show good 'run-
        off' into which a bypass graft
        may be plugged. The results
        of this kind of large vessel
        surgery are good.
        If your femoral pulse is present
        and of normal character, you
        have distal arterial disease.
        You may need a femoro-popliteal
        graft, an operation generally
        reserved for rest pain. The
        operative problems are greater
        and if things go badly wrong you
        are likely to lose the leg.

166.   a) Waxy pallor.
        b) Sensation loss.
        c) Temperature decrease.
        d) Muscle weakness→tenderness
           →rigidity (rigor mortis).
           (The limb will naturally be very
           painful, but this does not, of
           itself, indicate irreversible
           ischaemia.)

167.   What are the indications for
        arteriography in patients
        with intermittent claudication?

168.   Briefly summarise your understanding
        of the spectrum and likely out-
        come of intermittent claudication.

169.   List some of the important factors
        which influence the outcome of
        arterial surgery for chronic
        arterial occlusion.

167. Provided the patient is otherwise
     well, limiting claudication
     (less than 200 metres) which
     interferes with work or a
     satisfactory lifestyle. Thigh
     and buttock claudication indi-
     cate aorto-iliac disease.
     Symptoms range from mild to severe,
     associated with rest pain.
     Although 80% of patients stabilise
     and require no further treatment,
     15% - 20% have progressive disease
     and should be investigated.

168. Males > females.
     Usually a relatively benign
     condition. As various arteries
     silt up and occlude, exacerbations
     of intermittent claudication
     occur which then spontaneously
     improve over 2-3/12, giving a
     new claudication distance. Only
     about 15% progress to incipient
     gangrene.
     Surgery may be considered for the
     symptom of limiting claudication
     in the former, or for limb
     salvage in the latter.

169. It is better to operate on <u>localised</u>
     disease, in a <u>large</u> artery, <u>free</u>
     from calcification, in a <u>clean</u>
     field, in a relatively <u>young</u>,
     <u>non-diabetic</u>,patient who is in
     <u>good general</u> health, who has a
     <u>compelling</u> disability, who other-
     wise has a <u>bad</u> prognosis if left
     untreated. Reconstruction should
     be done by an <u>experienced</u> surgeon,
     and the patient must <u>stop smoking</u>.

170. Briefly describe the anterior compartment syndrome of the leg.

171. Aortic aneurysms are not that rare in the elderly. What features would lead you to consider referral for surgery?

172. What kinds of sympathectomy are there?

170.   Path.: ischaemic oedema of muscles
              of the anterior fascial
              compartment (tibia, fibula,
              deep fascia).
       Causes: trauma, fracture tib. and
              fib.; arterial occlusion;
              excess exercise; local
              bruising.
       Treatment: urgent surgical decom-
              pression by longitudinal
              fasciotomy.
       DD DVT: herein lies the danger.
              Anterior compartment syndrome
              may be mistaken for DVT and
              treated conservatively, with
              subsequent gangrene of the
              foot.

171.   1) Overt leaking; a near-absolute
          indication for surgery.
       2) Rapid enlargement: marked local
          tenderness+documented increase
          in diameter.
       3) Distal embolic disease: pieces
          of intramural thrombus embolising.
       4) Diameter on an ultrasound scan
          >5 cm (statistically more at
          risk of death from leakage than
          from an elective operation).
       5) Local or back pain.

172.   Surgical (division of the sympathetic
          chain).
       Chemical (local injection of phenol
          etc.).
       Pharmacological (ganglion blockers).
       Autosympathectomy, often only partial
          (diabetes).

173.   Describe the technique of taking
        blood out of the femoral vein.

174.   Is it inconsistent for a surgeon
        to refuse an elderly patient
        elective aortic aneurysm
        surgery, and yet be prepared
        to perform an emergency
        operation if it should leak?

175.   Do you think that it is ever easy
        or possible to inject drugs
        into the brachial artery
        instead of the basilic vein?
        Does this matter?

173.   The essential piece of information
        is that the vein lies <u>medial</u> to
        the artery.
        Place a finger over the artery and
        stab your needle firmly just
        medially as the vein passes over
        the bone (pubic ramus). Pull
        back the plunger to create a
        vacuum, and slowly withdraw the
        needle until it comes to lie in
        the femoral vein.
        Remember that the vein is often much
        more superficial than you imagine.
        When you remove the needle, maintain
        pressure on the puncture site for
        at least two minutes to reduce
        local bruising.

174.   No.
        In an old person the risk of death
        from an elective aneurysm
        operation (5-10% in the best
        hands) may well be comparable
        to the risk of death from it
        leaking or from other patholo-
        gies. Hence, no operation.
        Once the aneurysm has leaked the
        untreated mortality is 100%,
        and in this context, an opera-
        tive mortality of 65% is
        acceptable.

175.   Yes - surprisingly easy, especially
        in the emaciated elderly patient.
        After you have selected your 'vein' -
        <u>always</u> let down the cuff and
        ensure there is no pulse in it!
        After any i.v. injection, any
        discomfort should be felt in the
        upper arm and not in the hand.
        Inject a small quantity and ask
        whether the hand feels comfortable -
        if it does not - stop! Intra-
        arterial Diazepam may lead to
        peripheral gangrene - leave the
        needle in situ, and inject an
        antispasmodic down it (e.g.
        Papaverine 60 mg in saline).

176. Which patients might you select
      for referral for consideration
      for coronary artery by-pass
      surgery? Which is the key
      specialist investigation?

177. When assessing cardiac patients
      for possible referral for valve
      replacement is there any major
      difference between evolving
      mitral and aortic valve disease?

178. In chronic arterial insufficiency
      of the lower limb, does the
      pattern of symptoms give any
      clue as to the site of the
      lesion(s)?

176.   Youngish, i.e. < 65 years.
        Established crippling angina.
        'Crescendo angina'.
        The key investigation is coronary
            angiogram, which is not without
            risk, and is only worth doing
            if the patient is sufficiently
            fit to proceed to surgery. In
            general, 2 - 3 isolated lesions
            are suitable for by-pass surgery.
        The state of the myocardium itself
            is critical in the choice of
            patients for surgery.

177.   Yes.
        In mitral valve disease, the symptoms
            keep pace with severity, thus
            referral is indicated for disa-
            bility.
        In aortic valve disease, symptoms lag
            behind the haemodynamic disturbance
            and these people suddenly fall down
            dead. Thus referral is based on
            the physical signs before the
            symptoms become gross.

178.   Yes. A careful history may often
            give you a shrewd idea of the
            site of the block.
        Calf and foot pain only: suggests
            either
            (i) lower leg multiple blocks.
           (ii) superficial femoral artery
                occlusion + intact profunda.
          (iii) iliac occlusion with leg
                surviving on good collaterals.
        Thigh + leg + foot pain: suggests
            either
            SFA occlusion + profunda narrowing
            or aorto-iliac disease.
        Buttock pain is typical of proximal,
            aorto-iliac disease.

179.   Is there any need to investigate
        patients with transient
        cerebral ischaemic attacks,
        or is aspirin therapy the
        treatment of choice?

180.   Briefly outline the classic
        presentation of a leaking
        abdominal aortic aneurysm.

181.   Does a patient presenting with
        upper limb 'claudication'
        require any special tests?

179.   Clear-cut TIA's all should be
        investigated, initially with
        ultrasound imaging, if available,
        which selects those needing
        carotid angiography.
        40% are associated with carotid
        bifurcation disease.
        All tight stenoses should be
        considered for surgery, and many
        lesser lesions are suitable.

180.   Severe back pain with some abdominal
        pain + prostration.
        The patient feels very faint (due
        to retroperitoneal blood loss).
        Examination shows pallor, hypo-
        tension and a pulsatile abdominal
        mass + palpable femoral pulses.
        The abdominal mass may be surpris-
        ingly difficult to spot, it is
        the combination of severe back
        pain and hypovolaemia which is
        so suggestive.
        (Occasionally a leaking aneurysm
        may be misdiagnosed as ureteric
        colic.)

181.   Yes.
        The ability of the rich collateral
        circulations in the arm to
        compensate is so great that the
        symptom of claudication indicates
        gross disease likely to progress
        to overt gangrene.
        Look for both local factors (e.g.
        cervical rib, old fracture of
        clavicle) and general ones
        (giant cell arteritis).
        Early surgical intervention where
        appropriate may forestall further
        occlusions.

Bacteriology in Surgery

182.　　Dental extractions, urethral
　　　　　instrumentation, barium enema
　　　　　and sigmoidoscopy may give rise
　　　　　to which disease?
　　　　How could you prevent it?

183.　　Which organisms are usually grown
　　　　　from an ischiorectal abscess?
　　　　Is Ampicillin good treatment?

184.　　Does antibiotic prophylaxis have
　　　　　any place in amputations?

185.　　Which is the antibiotic of choice
　　　　　for a spreading streptococcal
　　　　　cellulitis?

182.   Bacterial endocarditis: all these
        procedures cause transient
        bacteraemia with Streptococci
        (viridans or faecal) and many
        other bacteria including
        Gram-negative organisms and
        Staphylococci which can lodge
        on damaged heart valves. Pre-
        vention involves giving anti-
        biotics starting with the
        premedication.

183.   Ischiorectal abscesses often grow
        organisms representing mixed
        faecal flora, i.e. mixed coli-
        forms + Bacteroides (anaerobes).
        Ampicillin has no activity
        against <u>Bacteroides</u> and is the
        wrong treatment.
        Ischiorectal abscesses require early
        incision and drainage.

184.   Yes - to protect against local sepsis
        and gas gangrene.
        Check the result of any culture swab
        from the limb.

        All above knee   )need benzyl
            amputations   )penicillin
        Most below knee   )prophylaxis with
            amputations   )premedication
            especially in   )against <u>Cl. Welchii</u>
            diabetics   )(perfringens),
                              <u>Staphylococci</u> and
                              other aerobes often,
                              and coliforms, rarely
                              require additional
                              antibiotic.

185.   Benzyl penicillin. Streptococci
        are always very sensitive.
        Erythromycin is a suitable
        alternative. Penicillin V
        ('oral' penicillin) is not well
        absorbed.

186.   a) When are prophylactic antibiotics
          used in biliary surgery?
       b) How long would you continue the
          prophylaxis in a patient making
          a good recovery?

187.   Which are the antibiotics of choice
       for the following post-operative
       severe chest infection?
       1) Pneumococcal (Str. pneumoniae)
       2) Haemophilus influenzae
       3) Staphylococcal

188.   Should head injury patients be
       given prophylactic antibiotics?

189.   Which organism is usually
       responsible for a breast
       abscess?
       Is its antibiotic sensitivity
       predictable?
       Should antibiotics be used?

186. a) All surgeons use prophylactic
          antibiotics when operating on
          the dilated obstructed biliary
          tree to avoid cholangitis and
          septicaemia.
          Most start antibiotics if they
          have to explore the common bile
          duct.
          Many start antibiotics when a
          cholecystectomy proves techni-
          cally difficult.
          Some use them for all chole-
          cystectomies, some never do.
          Cephalosporins and Ampicillin
          are both suitable.
      b) It is rarely necessary to give
          antibiotic prophylaxis for
          abdominal operations for more
          than 48 hours.

187. 1) Benzyl Penicillin.
      2) Amoxycillin.
      3) Flucloxacillin.

188. Only
      a) those with CSF leaks - to prevent
         meningitis.
      b) compound fracture - to prevent
         osteomyelitis, meningitis or
         abscess.
      c) retained foreign bodies,
         e.g. bullets.

189. Staphylococcus aureus
      90% of both G.P. and hospital
          cultures in Bristol are
          penicillin resistant, and
          Flucloxacillin is now the
          antibiotic of choice.
      Antibiotics can only be used
          in the early cellulitis stage.
          Once frank pus is present it
          requires drainage.

190.   Outline the principles governing
tetanus prophylaxis in a
patient with a heavily
contaminated wound.

190.　　1) Ascertain whether the patient
already has a level of immunity
(previous toxoid course + up-to-
date boosters).*A 3 dose course
of tetanus toxoid is effective
for at least 5 and probably 10
years: repeat injections of
unnecessary toxoid 'booster'
cause allergic reactions.

2) Estimate whether the nature of the
wound is likely to lead to tetanus,
e.g. crushed compound fracture of
the leg in manure heap - high risk.
Superficial scalp wound on the
dirty street - low risk.

3) Careful debridement of dead tissue
in all cases.

4) Gently dress the wound, do not
suture as a primary procedure.

5) Prophylactic Benzyl Penicillin
in all cases.

*6) High risk wound but currently
immunised patient⟶ Penicillin
(See(1) above).

*7) Low risk wound + currently
immunised patient⟶Penicillin
(See(1) above).

8) High risk wound + unimmunised
patient ⟶Penicillin + human
antitoxin.

9) Low risk wound + unimmunised
patient ⟶ Penicillin + toxoid
+ suitable advice concerning
observation, return to hospital
etc.

191.   Is the treatment of established
        tetanus easy?

192.   What is a subphrenic abscess?
        What is the 'catch phrase' about
            its diagnosis?

193.   Subphrenic abscess is a relatively
            uncommon, but serious complication
            of abdominal surgery. How would
            you diagnose it? How is it
            treated?

191.   No, it is a highly skilled, lengthy
        and difficult undertaking.
        The problems are:
        a) local surgery, antitoxin,
           debridement etc. to stop the
           production of more toxin.
        b) nurse away from noise,
           bustle etc.
        c) systemic Penicillin.
        d) Curarisation + elective
           ventilation for some weeks until
           the CNS recovers and tetanic
           spasms have ceased.
        e) the control of a labile auto-
           nomic nervous system that
           oscillates between hypo- and
           hyper-tension due to excitation
           of reflexes.
        f) keeping up the impetus of treatment
           during the long period with the
           goal of ultimate cure.

192.   Subphrenic = under (sub),
           the diaphragm (phrenic).
        Pus under the diaphragm on the
           right near the liver, on the
           left near the stomach and
           spleen.
        "Pus somewhere, pus nowhere = pus
           under the diaphragm".

193.   History of local pain + hiccough,
           + referral to shoulder tip.
        On examination - swinging pyrexia,
           relatively soft abdomen,
           pleural effusion.
        Chest x-ray - elevated hemidiaphragm +
           pleural effusion above it. Does
           not move on screening.
        Lung/liver scan - shows a gap
           between the two.
        Treatment - aspiration of pus and
           culture.
           Full antibiotic treatment.
           Formal abscess drainage is
           occasionally needed.
        The old concept that subphrenic sepsis
           must always be drained surgically is
           far less true nowadays with current
           antibiotics.

194.   How would you diagnose a post-
        operative pelvic abscess?

195.   How do you treat a pelvic abscess?

196.   Is spreading lymphangitis typically
        associated with streptococcal or
        staphylococcal infection?

194.   History of increasing lower
       abdominal discomfort 7 - 10
       days post-op.
       Unexplained diarrhoea or urinary
       frequency or ileus.
       Examination - swinging pyrexia.
                     In large abscess a
                     tender dull mass may
                     arise out of the pelvis.
                     Rectal and vaginal
                     examination - boggy
                     tender mass high up.

195.   Unless a) the patient is very toxic
                and ill and/or
              b) there is an unresolvable
                basic cause (e.g. burst
                anastomosis),
       the vast majority can be treated
          conservatively and encouraged
          to discharge p.r. or through
          the wound.
       Give mild analgesics.
       Use antibiotics only for generalised
          spreading problems.
       Repeated rectal examinations +
          occasional per-rectal incision.
       These abscesses usually discharge
          pus and the patient recovers.
       Many patients have subsequent
          problems with adhesive obstruction,
          chronic or recurrent sepsis and
          infertility (women).

196.   Streptococcal (Staphylococcal
          infections localise and form
          abscesses). Streptococci produce
          toxins (e.g. streptokinase and
          hyaluronidase)which lyse fibrin
          to increase the spread of
          infection, while Staphylococci
          tend to form abscesses.

197.   What is said to be the single
       most common cause of hospital
       acquired infection?

198.   Which six antibiotics should a
       surgeon take to a desert
       island?

199.   How would you treat a coliform
       septicaemia in a 70 year old
       man post-prostatectomy?

200.   How would you treat a group
       A beta-haemolytic streptococcal
       wound infection in a surgical
       patient?

197.   Urethral catheters.
       (40% of all hospital acquired
          infections are of the urinary
          tract: 75% of these are
          catheter related. Caveat: urinary
          tract infections are the easiest
          type of infection to detect and
          monitor and therefore may be
          statistically the commonest but
          not necessarily the most import-
          ant.)
       Treatment of catheter acquired
          bacteriuria with antibiotics is
          unnecessary unless the patient
          has symptoms. It is usually
          unsuccessful unless the catheter
          can be removed.

198.   Flucloxacillin/Penicillin/Amoxycillin/
          Gentamicin/Metronidazole/
          Cotrimoxazole. Cephalosporins are
          rarely required as 'first choice'
          antibiotics.

199.   Initial 'blind' therapy would
          probably include an aminoglycoside
          (Gentamicin) or a penicillin such
          as Ampicillin. Further therapy
          would be determined by the anti-
          biotic sensitivity results and
          the patient's progress. If
          Gentamicin is used, remember to
          monitor levels, as any degree of
          renal impairment may cause toxic
          accumulation of the drug.

200.   a) Give the patient Benzyl penicillin.
       b) Ensure the patient is barrier
          nursed (preferably in a side
          room) to prevent any spread of
          infection in the ward.

201. How would you treat a patient
developing severe diarrhoea
three days after a partial
gastrectomy?

201.   Check there is no physical cause
        for the diarrhoea (e.g. the
        patient becoming partially
        obstructed).
        Review the antibiotics the patient
        is receiving - Ampicillin is a
        well recognised cause of
        diarrhoea.
        Send a specimen of stool for culture
        for the common infectious patho-
        gens (e.g. Salmonella sp.).
        Consider the possibility of pseudo-
        membranous colitis. This is a
        condition in which previous
        antibiotic treatment (often with
        Clindamycin) causes overgrowth
        in the gut with <u>Clostridium
        difficile</u> which produces a toxin
        causing diarrhoea. Oral vancomycin
        is suitable treatment.

Cardiothoracic Surgery

202.   Why does blood not clot in the
        pleural cavity?

203.   What is an Ivor Lewis thoraco-
        abdominal resection?

204.   What is the differential diagnosis
        in an asymptomatic patient whose
        chest x-ray shows a well circum-
        scribed 'coin lesion' in the
        lung?

205.   Is radiotherapy indicated for a
        carcinoma of the oesophagus?

202.   It is defibrinated by the movement
       of heart and lungs. The quantities
       have to be large for the blood to
       clot.

203.   A two-stage operation to remove a
          tumour at the gastro-oesophageal
          junction/lower oesophagus.
       Stage I - abdominal laparotomy and
          mobilisation of the entire
          stomach, tumour and all.
       Stage II - after closure of the
          abdominal wound right lateral
          thoracotomy, drawing the
          oesophagus and stomach up into
          the chest, resection of the
          tumour and anastomosis of the
          oesophagus to intestine near the
          aortic arch.

204.   Bronchial carcinoma.
       Single pulmonary metatastic deposit.
       Benign bronchial adenoma.
       Bronchial hamartoma.
       Tb. focus.

205.   Yes.
       True squamous carcinoma of the
          oesophagus is usually radio-
          sensitive.
       The majority of lower 'oesophageal
          carcinomata' are gastric adeno-
          carcinomata involving the
          oesophagus - these are radio-
          resistant.

206.   Is there any major difference
       between the management of an
       intercostal drain tube when
       the whole lung has been removed,
       and when only a small part of it
       has been excised?

207.   What is haemoptysis?
       What is its differential diagnosis
           in a man of 65?

208.   Which are the key investigations
           in a man of 60 years
           presenting with recurrent
           haemoptyses?

209.   Should young children be discouraged
           from eating peanuts?
       If so, why?

206.   Yes.
        After pneumonectomy the hemithorax
            is empty and the drain is merely
            clamped.
        After lobectomy the hemithorax is
            still full because of the lung,and
            the drain is placed under a water
            seal to aid its expansion.
        If you connect the pneumonectomy
            drain to a water seal you will
            suck the mediastinum across into
            the empty hemithorax and the
            patient will collapse and may
            die!

207.   Haemoptysis is the coughing up of
            blood (haematemesis is vomiting
            it).
        1) Carcinoma of the bronchus.
        2) Pulmonary embolus.
        3) Tuberculosis.
        4) Bronchiectasis.
        5) Severe pulmonary oedema - really
           this is pink frothy sputum.
        6) No cause found - quite a common
           category.

208.   1) Chest x-ray (+laterals + tomograms
           if appropriate).
        2) Sputum, exfoliative cytology and
           Tb. culture.
        3) Bronchoscopy (+ bronchial
           brushings or biopsy).
        4) Mediastinoscopy with node biopsy
           where appropriate.

209.   Yes, there is a substantial risk of
            inhalation.
        Any child with a chest infection
            who admits to a cough and
            spluttering episode while eating
            peanuts should be regarded as
            having inhaled one until proved
            otherwise.
        Such patients need to be seen by an
            experienced clinician.
        Chest x-ray may show collapse, commonly
            right lower lobe. In most,
            bronchoscopy will be necessary.

210.   How should you remove a pleural
        drain?

211.   What is the first aid treatment
        of a penetrating chest injury
        leading to a hole in the
        chest wall that makes a
        sucking noise on respiration?

210. Make sure that the senior clinician has really authorised its removal.

If the patient is anxious, insert a butterfly needle and give a small amount of intravenous analgesia (say Pethidine 20 mg i.v.).

Always insist that a second person is present (e.g. a nurse) who can fetch help if difficulties develop.

Explain to the patient that you want him to perform a Valsalva manoeuvre (expiration against a closed glottis) as you withdraw the tube.

Remove the dressings. Check that there is a skin stitch in position to close the wound.

Cut the stitch retaining the tube.

Patient 'blows' Valsalva.

Nurse pulls out the tube in one steady movement and you snug down the skin stitch and cover the whole wound with gauze.

Once nurse has disposed of the tube, complete the knot and spray with plastic dressing.

Arrange a repeat chest x-ray for one hour's time.

211. Plug the hole with airtight bandage/lint/handkerchief etc.

Insert a drain connected to a valve/water seal as soon as practicable.

Transfer rapidly to hospital.

This is one occasion where a rapid ambulance ride is justified.

212.   What is a flail chest?
       How do you decide whether an
          injured patient has one?
       What is the initial treatment?

212.   A flail chest is thoracic cage
         instability caused by a series
         of fractures which disrupt the
         rigid hoop of rib-sternum-rib.
         Thus, on inspiration the ribs
         and sternum collapse inwards
         instead of expanding outwards,
         and the lungs do not change
         volume.
         Careful observation from the foot
         of the bed will reveal that the
         chest wall, or part of it
         (flail segment) moves paradoxi-
         cally with respiration.
         Palpation will confirm this.
         If the patient is unable to maintain
         oxygenation by his paradoxical
         respiratory efforts, he will
         become cyanosed and die.
         Emergency tracheal intubation and
         positive pressure ventilation
         is the treatment of choice.
         If there is only a flail segment
         the patient may become exhausted
         trying to avoid hypoxia, and
         need later, semi-elective
         intubation and PPV.
         There is a continuing risk of the
         fractured rib puncturing the
         lung and leading to a tension
         pneumothorax during such PPV.
         Many surgeons insert prophylactic
         pleural drains.

QUESTIONS CARDIOTHORACIC SURGERY 135

213. What is the first aid treatment in
the ward of an adult who is
choking to death with a piece
of food lodged in the larynx/
pharynx?

214. What is the first aid treatment of
acute laryngeal obstruction in
an infant?

213. 1) Give the patient a smart blow
         on the back hoping he will
         expel the lump.
      2) Try to remove the lump with your
         finger or forceps if available.
      3) If the patient is in extremis this
         is a difficult situation and you
         must appreciate that if the
         patient is about to die, however
         bad your treatment, it cannot
         make matters worse.
      Emergency tracheostomy is not for the
         amateur. You may cause so much
         bleeding that the patient inhales
         it into his cut trachea and drowns
         in his own gore!
      The least dangerous procedure is to
         take the biggest needle available,
         or better still a large i.v. cannula,
         and insert it into the gap between
         the thyroid cartilage (Adams apple)
         and the cricoid (i.e. through the
         cricothyroid membrane).
      If this fails, stick another one
         through the front of the trachea
         below this.
      This tiny tube will gain you enough
         time while your nurse secures
         senior help.

214. This is a desperately difficult
         situation.
      Slapping the back if a foreign body
         is suspected may help.
      Tracheostomy is especially hazardous
         in the young because the left
         innominate vein is higher than in
         an adult, and may cross the trachea
         above the sternal notch just where
         you wish to make the hole!
      Insert a large needle through the
         cricothyroid membrane.
      This small airway will give you a
         little time until expert help
         arrives.

215.   What is achalasia of the cardia?
       In whom does it occur?
       How is it treated?

216.   Is dysphagia commonly psychogenic,
       or not?

217.   Is the distinction between benign
       and malignant oesophageal
       stricture easy?

218.   Is intubation (e.g. Celestin tube)
       of a malignant oesophageal
       stricture often worth doing?

215. Achalasia of the cardia = cardio-
spasm = partial obstruction of
the distal oesophagus due to a
deficiency in the nervous
plexus.
Although thought to be of congenital
nature, it usually presents in
middle aged females.
A plain x-ray may show a fluid level
behind the heart, and a barium
swallow will outline the distal
oesophagus containing this fluid
with its typical sloped lower end.
Mild cases may respond to oesophageal
dilatation. The majority need a
myotomy (Heller's operation)
carried out either through the
chest or abdomen.

216. True dysphagia associated with a
feeling of food sticking is almost
always due to organic disease. It
is very dangerous indeed to
ascribe this symptom to hysteria
until you have seen at least two
normal barium swallow examinations
and endoscopies.

217. No.
Barium swallow examinations may be
misleading. Their function is to
demonstrate the stricture.
Diagnosis depends on (sometimes
repeated) endoscopic biopsy.

218. Yes, provided it is done with great
and gentle skill.
Death by dysphagia, unable to swallow
saliva, is degrading and ghastly.
Careful intubation either endoscopi-
cally or at (minor) operation will
enable the patient to swallow
saliva and semisolids until the
secondaries kill him.
If the surgeon punctures the growth
with the tube (very easy to do)
the patient will usually die from
sepsis within 24 hours.

219.   What advice must you give a patient
        going home with an oesophageal
        (Celestin) tube in situ?

220.   How do you pass a nasogastric (Ryles)
        tube?

221.   How do you know that a nasogastric
        tube is lying in the stomach?

219.   Eat semisolids only.
       Use a liquidiser for everything
          (the NHS will lend one).
       If food does stick, soda water will
          often clear it.
       If a blockage occurs, come back to
          Casualty.
       Sleep with many pillows (to reduce
          reflux).

220.   A confident approach is essential
          (and this only comes with
          practice!).
       More than any other procedure, this
          one is a personality clash
          between you and the patient. If
          he really thinks you believe that
          the tube is going down, it will.
       Give a little i.v. sedation (e.g. Diazepam
          5 mg i.v.).
       Sit the patient up holding a glass of
          water, lubricate the tip of the tube.
       Pass the N.G. tube through the nose
          until it reaches the pharynx.
       Make the patient take and hold a gulp
          of water in his mouth.
       Order him to swallow it, and chase the
          bolus down with your tube.

221.   1) Aspirated contents look gastric
             and turn litmus paper red.
       2) Water squirted down does not
             cause choking (tube down the
             trachea), and can be aspirated
             back.
       3) Blowing down the tube produces
             a bruit audible via stethoscope
             on the abdomen.
       4) Plain x-ray reveals N.G. tube tip
             below the diaphragm.

222.   How would you diagnose a spontaneous
        pneumothorax?
        How should it be treated?

223.   Is analysis of pleural effusion
        fluid often helpful?

222. The history is suggestive - sudden
marked pleuritic pain and short-
age of breath in a previously
fit thin young man.
The physical signs are difficult
unless the pneumothorax is gross:
absent/reduced breath sounds,
mediastinal shift away.
Plain chest x-ray - in expiration,
is conclusive. (The volume of
pneumothorax is fixed, the lung
volume varies. The pneumothorax
will be most obvious when the
latter is smallest, i.e. full
expiration.)
Treatment: use a large drain,
24 - 28F, i.e. the size of your
little finger.
a) minor pneumothorax - observation
only.
b) major pneumothorax - large I.C. tube
and suction. One drain should
be adequate.
if it   i) fails to reinflate)
           ii) continues to   ) refer
               bubble ++   ) to
          iii) deflates on ceasing) chest
               suction   ) unit
           iv) recurs   )

223. Yes, frequently.
Clear serous fluid, low protein =
transudate, e.g. heart failure.
Turbid, odourless, slightly blood
stained = malignant exudate -
cytology confirms.
Turbid, smelly, purulent = infected
effusion⟶ empyema = lung or
subdiaphragmatic sepsis.
Blood stained, small amount = pulmonary
infarct.

224.   On the tenth post-operative day your
        cholecystectomy patient develops
        marked left pleuritic pain and
        breathlessness. What complication
        do you suspect? How do you diagnose
        it? What is the initial treatment?

225.   In a large teaching hospital, how
        might a major life threatening
        pulmonary embolus be managed in
        a young adult?

226.   Cardiopulmonary bypass (the 'pump')
        has become a routine procedure
        in cardiac centres.
        Briefly state:
        1. what the machine does?
        2. how does this help the operating
            surgeon?

224.   Pulmonary embolism.
        History: sudden onset of pleuritic
            pain and breathlessness. Ask
            about haemoptysis.
        Examination: increased respiratory
            rate + normal breath sounds
            $\pm$ pleural rub.

        Signs of D.V.T. in legs.
        Signs of right heart strain,
            raised J.V.P., IIIrd sound.
        Tests: E.C.G. shows right heart
            strain. Chest x-ray normal or
            decreased vascular markings.
        Treatment: Heparin, oxygen.

225.   1) Full heparinisation.
        2) Emergency pulmonary arteriogram
            to establish diagnosis and/or
            ventilation/perfusion radio-
            active scan of lung.
        3) Either - intra-arterial Streptokinase
            down the pulmonary catheter
            or
            open embolectomy or cardiopulmonary
            bypass.
        4) Venogram to identify embolus source $\pm$
            caval surgery.

226.   1. Through cannulae the pump takes all
           the (low pressure) blood from the
           S.V.C. and I.V.C., extracts CO_2 and
           adds O_2 in a disposable plastic
           exchanger, removes bubbles, and
           finally returns the blood at
           arterial pressure to the arch of
           the aorta. This perfuses the rest of
           the body including the myocardium via
           the coronary arteries.
        2. The heart becomes empty of blood.
           By cooling or electric shock it can
           be made still for several hours.
           The heart can be opened and delicate
           unhurried surgery to valves etc.
           carried out in a clear, motionless,
           dry field.

227.   Emergency embolectomy for massive
        pulmonary embolism has sometimes
        been advocated. Once the patient
        is successfully 'on bypass' the
        life threatening thrombus can be
        extracted from the pulmonary
        artery virtually at leisure.
        How long do you think it takes in a
        well organised unit to establish
        bypass?

228.   What are the three main methods of
        treating pulmonary embolism and
        their indication?

227.   Assuming that you have enough
       compatible blood to prime the
       pump (2 units), that everyone
       is ready, and that the operation
       is straightforward, at least
       half an hour from induction of
       anaesthesia.

228.   a) Anticoagulants - minor emboli
          without haemodynamic disturbances.
       b) Thrombolytics - major emboli with
          haemodynamic disturbance not
          life threatening within 12-24 hr.
       c) Embolectomy - serious cardio-
          vascular disturbance with death
          likely before other treatment
          can be effective.

Endocrine Surgery

229.   Your patient has a solitary nodule
        palpable in the thyroid and a
        scan shows that it is 'hot' with
        suppression of the rest of the
        gland. Is this likely to be
        malignant?

230.   What instructions should be given to
        a patient about to commence a course
        of Carbimazole for hyperthyroidism?

231.   What E.N.T. investigation should
        usually be performed prior to
        any thyroid operation?

232.   Why are pre-operative x-rays taken
        of the neck in a patient about
        to undergo surgery for goitre?
        Which views are commonly requested?

233.   What are the specific early compli-
        cations of thyroidectomy?

229.   No. It is excessively unusual for
        hot nodules to be malignant, they
        are usually benign adenomata.
        They should be excised by hemi-
        thyroidectomy and the prognosis
        is good.

230.   This drug must be taken 8 hourly and
        not 'three times a day'. The
        common cause of treatment failure
        is irregular timing of the drug.
        The major (rare) side effect is bone
        marrow depression. Ask the patient
        to report any sore throats or
        malaise, and do a F.B.C. if they do.

231.   Indirect laryngoscopy (an out-patient
        procedure).
        Up to 3% of the population have an
        asymptomatic partial or complete
        cord palsy. If any question of
        operative recurrent laryngeal
        nerve damage arises, this base-
        line information may be of great
        value.

232.   To check for tracheal deviation or
        compression which is usually
        symptomless but a warning sign
        that respiratory obstruction might
        develop post-operatively. A.P.,
        lateral and thoracic inlet views
        are usually requested. A multi-
        nodular goitre may show calcifi-
        cation.

233.   1st day: reactionary haemorrhage.
                 recurrent laryngeal nerve
                   palsy or temporary paresis.
                 thyroid crisis.
        2nd-3rd day: hypocalcaemia due to
                 parathyroid damage. Presents
                 as circumoral tingling,
                 Chvostek's and Trousseau's
                 signs positive.
        4th day: wound infection.

234. You are called urgently to see your
     patient five hours after thyroid-
     ectomy. She is distressed,
     frightened, and breathless with
     a swollen neck and tachycardia.
     What should you do?

235. What mnemonic summarises the present-
     ation of hypercalcaemia?

236. Is O.P.D. clinic follow up of
     thyroidectomy patients worth-
     while? What is the minimum that
     should be done at each visit?

234. The diagnosis is either tracheal
      compression due to reactionary
      haemorrhage or acute thyroid
      crisis.
      Sit the patient up: start 100%
      oxygen by MC mask: give a small
      amount of sedation, e.g. Diazepam
      5 mg i.v.
      If the pulse rate is below 150/min.,
      you have a little time.
      Think - hard: the two conditions are
      very different.
      Thyroid crisis looks like thyrotoxi-
      cosis in excelsis, i.e. tachycardia,
      restlessness, pyrexia, tremor. It
      responds to more Diazepam
      + Propranolol i.v.
      Tracheal compression looks like
      strangulation: breathlessness,
      stridor, cyanosis, etc.
      Cut the stitches and clips and the
      deep vertical layer of stitches
      in the strap muscles, evacuate
      the clot and place a light pack
      in situ.
      If the stridor continues you need an
      anaesthetist, and the patient will
      need to go back to theatre anyway.

235. Stones, bones and abdominal groans.

236. Yes, to identify late onset hypo-
      thyroidism.
      Take a rapid thyroid history.
      Check that the original histology
      was benign.
      Check the patient's weight.
      Look at the neck.
      Take the pulse. If it is between 65
      and 95 per min. the patient is
      almost certainly euthyroid.
      Routine blood tests are costly and
      unnecessary if the patient is
      clinically euthyroid and feels
      well.

237. List the classic symptoms of
      hyperthyroidism.

238. On admission for elective thyroid
      surgery, is the thyroid status
      of the patient important?

239. What is the differential diagnosis
      of a diffuse firm thyroid
      swelling in a woman of 35?

237.   Feeling hot, insensitivity to cold.
        Weight loss.
        Tremor.
        Diarrhoea.
        Menstrual upset - usually oligo-
            menorrhoea.
        Mental agitation/anxiety.
        Tachycardia, palpitations.
        Eye changes - protuberance, double
            vision, discomfort.
        Warm sweaty hands.

238.   Yes.
        To operate on an uncontrolled
            hyperthyroid gland is to risk
            the life-threatening complication
            of acute thyroid crisis. All
            thyroid patients should have had
            thyroid hormone levels recorded, so
            check these.
        Make a clinical assessment of hypo/
            hyper/euthyroid status. Euthyroid
            patients, having had no therapy
            need no special measures.
        Controlled toxic patients require
            Propranolol + Diazepam cover
            (Lugol's iodine is seldom used
            now).
        Uncontrolled toxic patients -
            consider postponing operation
            unless there are compelling
            indications for what is now urgent
            (and not elective) surgery.

239.   1) Hashimoto's Disease - gland is
              rubbery.
        2) Anaplastic carcinoma - gland is
              woody hard.
        3) Medullary carcinoma - rare (C cells).
        4) Graves' Disease - the diffusely
              enlarged thyroid is accompanied
              by gross thyrotoxicosis).

240.   List the renal changes that may occur
        in hyperparathyroidism.

241.   How does their position allow you to
        distinguish between thyroglossal
        cyst, thyroglossal fistula,
        branchial cyst, branchial fistula
        and pharyngeal pouch?

242.   How may a goitre cause acute
        respiratory obstruction?

243.   What are the main causes of post-
        operative respiratory
        obstruction after thyroidectomy?

244.   When you examine a patient with a
        goitre, what are the main clinical
        features that you must establish
        that will affect how you further
        investigate and treat the patient?

240.   1) Nephrocalcinosis (bilateral).
        2) Renal - ureteric stones (may be
               unilateral).
        Which may lead to:-
        3) Chronic renal failure.
        4) Hypertension.

241.   Thyroglossal cyst: Always in midline.
            Usually between hyoid bone and
            thyroid cartilage. Protrusion of
            tongue makes cyst move.
        Thyroglossal fistula: Midline track
            associated with the above.
        Branchial cyst: Lies near angle of
            jaw in upper third of neck partly
            behind sternomastoid.
        Branchial fistula: Lies on anterior
            border of sternomastoid and may
            communicate with branchial cyst.
        Pharyngeal pouch: Lies in middle
            third of neck, deep in posterior
            triangle.
            Can be emptied into pharynx by
            firm pressure.

242.   Spontaneous haemorrhage (into a
            degenerating nodule) within the
            thyroid, and this may be retro-
            sternal.

243.   Damaged recurrent laryngeal nerve(s)
            (cords adduct).
        Tracheal collapse - tracheomalacia.
        Post-operative haematoma (leading to
            venous congestion and laryngeal
            oedema).
        Laryngeal oedema.

244.   a) Goitre - multinodular or single
                        lump.
                     ? palpable local lymph nodes.
                     ? recurrent laryngeal
                        nerve paresis.
        b) Thyroid status - hypo/hyper/eu-
                        thyroid.

245. List the clinical features of
      Cushing's syndrome, briefly.

246. Once you have established a diagnosis
      of Cushing's syndrome you need
      to establish its cause. List
      four different sources for the
      excess glucocorticoids.

247. Hormone secreting tumours of the
      pancreas may give rise to three
      types of endocrine disorder.
      Name these.

245.   Cushingoid facies: moon face, acne,
          striae, bruising etc.
       Buffalo neck hump; weight gain;
          muscle wasting and weakness.
       Hypertension; amenorrhoea;
          susceptibility to infections;
          ...... and many more!

246.   a) Iatrogenic (Gk iater = physician)
          steroid treatment,
          e.g. prednisolone. This has
          made Cushing's syndrome a
          common condition.
       b) Overproduction by the adrenal(s):
          hyperplasia, tumour.
       c) Excess pituitary ACTH: Pituitary
          tumour.
       d) Ectopic ACTH production: carcinoma
          or adenoma of bronchus is the
          commonest.

247.   a) Hypoglycaemic attacks from
          insulinoma.
       b) Intractable peptic ulceration
          from gastrinoma (Zollinger-
          Ellison Syndrome).
       c) Watery diarrhoea from VIPoma
          (non α non β cell tumour).

E.N.T. Surgery

248. In taking the history from a patient
     with a parotid swelling, what
     particular questions should be
     asked?

249. Give the differential diagnosis of a
     subcutaneous swelling tucked
     behind the lobe of the ear.

250. What are the commoner causes of
     parotid swelling?

251. You are asked by your examiner to
     feel a lump in a patient's neck.
     What should you always do apart
     from looking at and feeling the
     neck before reporting your
     findings?

248.   1) How long has he noticed the
          swelling?
       2) Has it changed in size, and if so,
          slowly or rapidly and or in
          relation to food?
       3) Is it painful, at rest or during
          or after chewing/eating?
       4) Is there any discharge of saliva
          or pus into the mouth?
       5) Has he noticed facial weakness?
       6) Has he received any treatment for
          it recently or in the past?

249.   1) Parotid gland or tumour   )
       or   )VAST
       2) Lymphadenopathy - non-specific)MAJOR-
          inflammatory or specific or   )ITY
          secondary carcinoma   )
       3) Sebaceous cyst   )
       4) Inclusion dermoid   )OCCASIONALLY
       5) Lipoma   )
       6) Histiocytoma   )

250.   a) mumps (usually children, but
          occasionally in adults).
       b) neoplasm benign or malignant.
       c) calculi.
       d) parotitis of other aetiologies -)
          Mikulicz syndrome due to   )
          sarcoid/reticulosis/   )Rarer
          Sjogren/Tb.   )
       e) drug induced   )

251.   The patient should be examined to
          exclude carcinoma of the mouth.
          tongue, upper respiratory and
          upper alimentary tracts.

252. What structures should you be able
        to identify on indirect laryngoscopy?

253. What conditions in <u>infancy</u> may cause
        stridor?

254. Do benign neoplasms occur in the
        larynx?

255. Clearly not all patients reporting
        'loss of voice' require immediate
        investigation for laryngeal
        pathology. What simple rule of
        thumb is usually applied to the
        situation?

256. What simple bedside tests can
        indicate the presence of a
        recurrent laryngeal palsy or
        paresis?

252. Lower pole of the tonsils; posterior
      third of tongue; valleculae;
      epiglottis; ary-epiglottic folds;
      piriform fossae; hypopharynx;
      ventricular bands; vocal cords;
      upper tracheal rings.

253. 1) Congenital laryngeal stridor
         (laryngo-malacia).
      2) Congenital subglottic stenosis.
      3) Laryngeal haemangioma.
      4) Laryngeal web.
      5) Laryngotracheobronchitis.
      N.B. Epiglottitis causes supra
         laryngeal obstruction and noisy
         breathing but not true stridor.

254. Yes.
      Papilloma (about 85%)
      Adenoma   )
      Chondroma) about 5% each
      Angioma, neurofibroma (less than 5%)

255. Patients whose hoarseness of voice
      has persisted for over three
      weeks require E.N.T. referral
      and assessment including indirect
      laryngoscopy.

256. Ask the patient to give a good cough
      (which requires closure of the
      glottis).
      Try to elicit a Valsalva manoeuvre.
      Request the patient to sing a scale
      (difficult if one nerve has been
      paralysed).
      Listen for breath escape during
      speech.
      Test how far the patient can count
      in one breath (i.e. one, two,
      three, four etc.).

257. As an alternative to emergency trache-
     ostomy, the thrusting of several
     wide bore needles through which
     structure may temporarily relieve a
     complete upper respiratory tract
     obstruction?

258. Headache, oedematous eyelids, rigors
     and a septic focus on the nose are
     pathognomonic of what?

259. What are the commoner causes of
     ulceration of the tongue?

260. What are the indications for
     tonsillectomy?

261. Name three ways in which a naso-
     pharyngeal carcinoma may often
     present.

262. State briefly the aim of radical
     neck dissection.

257.   The cricothyroid membrane.

258.   Cavernous sinus thrombosis.

259.   Common: aphthous, trauma from teeth
           or dentures, viral ulceration.
       Less common: carcinoma, syphilis,
           leukoplakia, Behcet's.
       Rare: Pemphigoid, Tb, median
           rhomboid glossitis.

260.   a) Absolute: post-quinsy (abscess),
             after an interval of about six
             weeks.
             Suspected malignancy.
       b) Relative: recurrent acute tonsillitis
             causing time lost from school,
             other complications of large
             tonsils: recurrent otitis media,
             bronchitis, exacerbations of
             psoriasis.
             streptococcal carrier unresponsive
             to antibiotics.
             cor pulmonale in children due to
             large tonsils.

261.   1) enlarged cervical node.
       2) conductive deafness as a result
             of invasion of the Eustachian
             tube and consequent to middle
             ear effusion.
       3) cranial nerve palsy.

262.   To clear as far as possible the
       lymph nodes draining the head
       and neck region which may contain
       metastatic tumour, while retaining
       vital structures.

263. How can you control epistaxis
     (nose bleed)?

264. Why should you treat epistaxis in
     the elderly as an emergency?

265. Which E.N.T. clinical signs support
     the suspicion of a fractured base
     of the skull?

266. What is a cauliflower ear? How is
     it caused and treated?

267. What is a positive Rinné test?

268. Is it positive in sensori-neural
     deafness?

263.   1) Digital pressure.
       2) Nasal cautery (electric not
          chemical).
       3) Nasal packing.
       4) Ligation of arteries (rarely
          needed).

264.   Because of the risk of major blood
       loss and rapid cardiovascular
       collapse.

265.   1) C.S.F. rhinorrhoea or otorrhoea.
       2) Haemotympanum with an intact drum.
          (Blood in the middle ear with
          dark blue drum.)
       3) Blood at the external auditory
          meatus in the absence of other
          obvious injury to the ear by
          trauma or explosion.

266.   An unsightly deformed pinna and
       concha, due to organised haematoma
       in the subperichondrial space,
       following trauma to the external
       ear. Ideally it should be prevented
       by immediate drainage of the haema-
       toma after the trauma. This is
       seldom done, with the resultant
       distortion of the ear which is
       practically impossible to correct
       later.

267.   The ability to hear a tuning fork held
       close to the meatus when it is no
       longer heard when placed on the
       mastoid process.

268.   Yes.

269.   How are prominent ears corrected?

270.   What is a myringotomy? When is it
          indicated? What advice should
          be given to parents of children
          who have just had one performed?

271.   What complications may arise from a
          chronically discharging ear with
          cholesteatoma?

269.   By one of numerous operative techniques,
       most of which employ 'the breaking
       of the helical spring'. The peri-
       chondrium and or underlying carti-
       lage on the lateral aspect of the
       pinna is abraded or incised
       allowing the ear to lie back
       against the scalp. The ear is
       then fixed in the corrected position
       with sutures with or without excision
       of postauricular skin.

270.   Myringotomy is an incision, usually
       radial of the tympanic membrane.
       It is indicated when fluid is
       present or is suspected in the
       middle ear. The ear should be
       protected from water until the
       drum has healed (i.e. no swimming
       for several days).

271.   1.   Deafness.
       2.   Intracranial sepsis (meningitis/
            cerebral abscess).
       3.   Facial palsy.
       4.   Vertigo from erosion of the
            lateral semi-circular canals.
       5.   Lateral sinus thrombosis leading
            to septicaemia.
       6.   Carcinoma of the ear.

Gynaecology in Surgery

272.   When does an ectopic pregnancy
        usually rupture?

273.   You are tired, overworked and at the
        end of a long day you are asked
        to see a 17 year old girl in
        Casualty with mild abdominal pain
        who 'should have gone to her G.P.'
        What are the pitfalls?

274.   You examine a 30 year old lady in
        Casualty with abdominal pain and
        discover a dull mass arising out
        of the pelvis to the umbilicus.
        How do you proceed?

272.   Rupture commonly occurs about 6-10
       weeks after the L.M.P., i.e.
       there is usually a history of
       one 'missed' or 'late' period,
       or of irregular bleeding.

273.   This is a classic 'custard pie'
       situation. Be careful. Because
       you are annoyed, you are likely
       to make mistakes.
       The absolute minimum is a reasonable
       abdominal history and a menstrual
       history, together with a careful
       examination, including rectal and
       vaginal examination. The great
       danger is that you will miss an
       ectopic pregnancy or appendicitis.

274.   You will have taken a full history
       before examining her and will
       know whether she is likely to be
       pregnant. If she is, immediate
       joint consultation between senior
       gynaecologist and surgeon is
       needed.
       The differential diagnosis is bladder,
       ovarian cyst or a rarity.
       Pass a catheter. If the mass disappears,
       it was bladder.
                       If the mass remains,
       repeat the pelvic examination.
       Plain x-rays and ultrasound will
       confirm an ovarian cyst.
       Refer to a gynaecologist, keeping at
       the back of your mind the idea
       that although she happens to have
       an ovarian cyst the abdominal pain
       may still be due to other pathology
       such as appendicitis, urinary
       infection etc.

275.   Do young girls with abdominal pain
often lie to you about whether
they might be pregnant?

276.   Describe the clinical presentation
of a twisted ovarian cyst of
moderate size.

275.   Yes, frequently because of the
        presence of their mother during
        your consultation.
        Housemen are often amazed at the
        way a more senior clinician can
        worm out this information.
        Take the history with the mother
        present, but conduct the examin-
        ation in the presence only of a
        nurse   which gives you the chance
        to ask more questions. Prior to
        rectal examination, careful
        scrutiny will reveal whether a
        hymen is present, if not, whether
        a one or two finger vaginal
        examination is possible. Few
        girls will lie about sexual
        experience during a vaginal
        examination because they imagine
        that the doctor can tell (he
        can't!).
        If you remain suspicious of pregnancy,
        remember the adage that it is
        usually safer to 'assume all
        women are pregnant until proved
        otherwise'.

276.   There may be a past history of
        previous minor episodes of pain.
        There has often been no menstrual
        irregularity.
        Iliac fossa pain coming on over
        $\frac{1}{2}$ hour and radiating to the
        inner thigh below the inguinal
        ligament, often colicky in nature.
        Vomiting may occur, but is not
        persistent.
        Examination reveals a generally soft
        abdomen with tenderness and
        guarding low in the iliac fossa.
        P.V. there is either a tender mass
        in a fornix or this area is so
        tender that accurate palpation
        is impossible.
        Treatment is operative excision of
        the cyst.

277.   When a female patient is admitted
       for elective or emergency
       surgery, why is it important
       to discover what type of contra-
       ception she uses?

278.   How do you distinguish between ovulatory
       pain, dysmenorrhoea and acute
       appendicitis?

279.   You are a G.P. and see a 25 year
       old lady in your surgery 26 weeks
       pregnant with a six hour history
       of marked abdominal pain. What
       should you do?

277.   Patients taking the contraceptive
        pill have an increased risk of
        thrombo-embolism after surgery.
        Most procedures should be
        covered by 'miniheparin'
        (Heparin 5,000 units sc t.d.s)
        prophylaxis, or alternative
        prophylactic measures.

278.   This can be difficult. The key
        lies in a careful history and
        repeated examinations.
        Dysmenorrhoea is premenstrual or
        menstrual, ovulatory pain occurs
        mid-cycle (12-14 days premenstru-
        ally).
        Admit the patient and re-examine her
        when she is comfortable in bed,
        every one to two hours until the
        diagnosis becomes plain.
        Remember that if you are going to be
        wrong it is better to remove a
        normal appendix in error than to
        leave an inflamed one to burst.

279.   Refer her to hospital immediately.
        Marked abdominal pain that does
        not disappear with minor analgesics
        is abnormal. Diagnosis of the
        acute pregnant abdomen can be
        exceedingly difficult for even the
        most experienced. The patient's
        best hope is to be seen as early as
        possible by the hospital doctors
        who are going to have to decide
        whether to operate or not.

280.   You are called urgently to Casualty
       to see a girl of 20 years,
       'collapsed', with a ruptured
       ectopic pregnancy. When you arrive
       you find a pale, anxious,
       hypovolaemic woman who appears in
       extremis. As H.S. what are your
       priorities?

280. 1. The priority is to establish a
        good i.v. line to give her
        fluids while preparations
        are made for operation.
        If you are confident of your
        own abilities, get on with
        this and ask others to inform
        your seniors.
        If you are 'not much good at
        drips' (yet), this is no time
        to start learning. Ask the
        C.O. to start the drip, and
        you contact your Registrar
        and duty anaesthetist.
        Have only two attempts at a
        percutaneous drip before
        proceeding to cut down. The
        long saphenous vein at the
        ankle is the easiest. Once
        you have exposed it, you can
        stab it with your standard
        needle-cannula under vision.

     2. Take 30 ml blood from the
        femoral vein if necessary for
        cross-matching 4 units.

     3. Start your drip with saline and
        then change to a plasma
        expander - PPF, haemocel. In
        dire straits, use O-neg.

     4. By now you have to have senior help
        because operation is needed to
        save this girl's life. If you
        are having difficulty in
        finding the right person,
        remember any surgeon will
        suffice - orthopaedic,
        urological, even plastic!

Haematology in Surgery

281.   From the moment you decide you want
        to transfuse a patient with blood,
        how long does it take for the
        laboratory to provide you with an
        appropriate bottle?
        a) routinely
        b) urgently
        c) dire emergency?

282.   How much O negative blood do you think
        an average district general hospital
        carries in stock at any one time?

281.   Allow five minutes for you to   )
          take the blood, label the   )
          bottle, complete the forms   )
          and telephone the Blood Bank.)
       Porterage.   ) $\frac{1}{2}$ hr.
       1/4 hr. for the laboratory to   )
          separate serum and ABO group)
          and Rhesus type.   )
       Then
       a) standard x-match = $\frac{1}{2}$ hr. + 2 hrs.
             cross match donor cells vs.
             recipient serum - complete Ab
                              cold Ab
                              incomplete Ab.
       b) urgent = $\frac{1}{2}$ hr. + $\frac{1}{2}$ hr. (cross match
             accelerated using centrifuge
             'spin' techniques, for Ab
             detection) - complete Ab
                          incomplete Ab.
       c) dire emergency (rare) = 0 + 0 -
             immediate issue screened O-ve.
             "universal donor" blood.

282.   Only about 5 units screened for
          atypical Ab.
       All blood issued from transfusion
          centres, is 'screened'.

283.   What is a "transfusion reaction"?
        How would you know your patient was
            having one?
        What action should you take to treat
            the patient and diagnose the cause?

283. "Transfusion reaction" is usually
      taken to mean a great or small
      immunological response by the
      recipient to incompatible blood.
      The expression may also include
      minor pyrogenic reaction to
      components of compatible blood
      (e.g. white cell antigens).
Clinical: new bottle of blood
      recently put up. Relatively
      sudden (5 - 30 mins.) onset of
      pyrexia, rigors, backache ± rash,
      tachycardia.
      May proceed (rarely) via broncho-
      spasm ──→ angioneurotic oedema ──→
      (even more rarely) anaphylaxis
      ──→ death.
      A major ABO mis-match produces
      complete vasomotor collapse.
Treatment: remove blood + giving set,
      and replace with saline and new
      set.
      Antihistamine (e.g. Chlorpheniramine
      25 mg i.v.)
      Hydrocortisone 100 mg i.v.
      (only in extremis - Adrenaline
      1:1000 i.m. 0 - 0.5 ml slowly).
      Minor analgesics.
N.B. Our expert considers that minor
      episodes of pyrexia only can often
      be ignored quite safely. Too many
      bottles of blood are wasted by
      being taken down at the first
      flicker of temperature.
Diagnosis: inform the Blood Bank.
      Send them the suspected blood +
      giving set; a new specimen of
      clotted + sequestrene blood,& urine
      sample.

284.   What is the commonest cause of a
        mis-matched blood transfusion?

285.   What is the lowest level of platelets
        usually regarded as adequate in a
        patient about to undergo a routine
        major surgical operation?

286.   What are the main features of <u>gross</u>
        acute disseminated intravascular
        coagulation?

287.   Where might you expect to find
        splenunculi at operation?
        Why do they matter?

284.   Clerical error in the labelling of
       the donor blood either at
       venesection, in the laboratory
       or at the recipient's bedside.
       This accounts for ¾ of all
       mis-matches.

285. $100 \times 10^9/1$ ($100,000/mm^3$)
       Below this some thought needs to be
       given to the relative risks of
       bleeding, transfusion and
       operation.

286.   This is a grave and often fatal
          development.
       Haemorrhage - often first noticed
          as persistent oozing from vene-
          puncture sites and surgical
          incisions.
       Circulatory collapse.
       ± Multiple microthrombi - cerebral
          coma, convulsions, psychosis.
          Renal - oliguria/anuria.
       (The thrombotic complications may
          also sometimes occur on their own.)

287.   Near the hilum of the spleen; in the
          omentum, occasionally elsewhere.
       If retained after therapeutic
          splenectomy, they may hypertrophy
          and restore some splenic function.

Miscellaneous and Nursing

288.   How do you cope with a patient who
        insists on taking his own
        discharge against medical
        advice?

289.   What administrative action should
        you take when one of your
        patients dies in hospital?

288.   Recognise that this is a tricky
         situation that may have later
         repercussions.
       Insist on a witness, preferably an
         experienced nurse, and inform
         your Registrar.
       The actual decision, stripped of
         histrionics, is remarkably
         simple: either
       a) the patient is clinically insane
         and a danger to himself and
         others, in which case he must
         be certified and then forced
         to stay, which means sedation.
         or
       b) he is in your view, misguided
         and must be permitted to leave.
         Ask him to sign the 'own
         discharge' form. If he refuses,
         record this in the notes.
       Always make a written record in the
         case-notes, countersigned by your
         witness and then inform your
         Registrar.

289.   Between 9.00 a.m. and 10.00 p.m.
         telephone your Consultant. After
         all, the person was his patient
         and not yours. If the patient
         dies at night, telephone first
         thing next morning. Ask permission
         to issue a death certificate
         + autopsy.
       Likewise telephone the patient's
         general practitioner. A good
         family doctor will usually check
         that all is well with a surviving
         spouse.
       Inform your Registrar.
       Follow the hospital policy for
         informing the next of kin.

290.   What should you do when a G.P. rings
       you as the duty H.S. requesting
       admission for a patient, and you
       suspect that admission is
       inappropriate?

291.   Do you have the authority as a
       pre-registration house surgeon
       to discharge patients home?

292.   Who decides whether to refer a
       patient's death to H.M. Coroner?

290.   Recognise that all G.P.'s will be
        much older and more experienced
        than you and will resent being
        subjected to examination style
        inquisition, particularly if you
        end by saying "No'."
        Try to appreciate that the social
        circumstances of a patient may
        necessitate temporary admission
        for an intrinsically minor illness.
        Either insist on seeing the patient
        in Casualty first, or take the
        G.P.'s number and tell him politely
        that your Registrar will ring him
        directly.

291.   Whatever the precise legal position,
        in practice you do not.
        The two most irrevocable management
        steps to take for a surgical
        patient are to operate, or to
        send him home.
        You must not do either without the
        direct authority of your immediate
        superior.

292.   The Consultant Surgeon or, only when
        he is on leave, his deputy. As,
        sadly, you are likely to observe,
        a quite disproportionate amount
        of mayhem is caused by housemen
        who fail to follow this simple
        dictum and erroneously either do,
        or do not, report cases. At worst,
        you may be summoned to appear in
        Court before the Coroner for a
        public humiliation which provides
        absorbing copy for the local press!

293.   What should you do when a patient
       starts to make vitriolic
       complaints about you to your
       face?

294.   What should you do if you think
       you have made some serious
       clinical error of commission
       or omission?

293.   Do not be too surprised. However
       good a doctor you think you are,
       this is certain to happen to
       you at least once during your
       housejob.
       Never lose your temper, and do not
       become a party to a mid-ward
       harangue.
       Withdraw smartly - gracefully if
       possible - if not, just withdraw.
       Return promptly with a senior nurse.
       Pull the curtains around the bed
       and start again.
       If you cannot defuse the situation
       within five minutes, retreat.
       Tell your superiors who will know
       how to cope.
       Always make a written record, signed
       by your witness, in the case-notes.
       Substantial complaints or allegations
       must be referred to your Consultant
       without delay.

294.   The golden rule is to confess at once
       to your superiors.
       It is fair to say that virtually
       nothing you can do will shock or
       surprise an experienced Senior
       Registrar or Consultant. If you
       never make any mistakes, you
       should have his job!
       Once the facts are in the open, you
       may be certain the senior members
       will rally round to extract the
       coals from the fire. If they
       don't know what has happened, they
       cannot help.
       You can rest assured that in their own
       past they each have some murky
       memories every bit as bad as your
       recent sin.

295.   If your patient dies soon after an
       operation and it is plain that
       the Coroner will need to be
       informed, are there any special
       instructions you need to give
       the nurses regarding the laying
       out of the body?

296.   Do you really think that bad news
       should ever be given to relatives
       over the telephone? If so, are
       there any important guidelines to
       follow?

297.   Are there any guidelines for how
       you should go about breaking
       bad news to the relatives of
       your patients in hospital?

295. Yes. All apparatus (e.g. endo-
tracheal tube, catheter, drip
cannulae) must be left in situ.
Their correct positioning may
later become an issue at an
inquest.

296. In theory, no; but what are you to
do when your R.T.A. patient's
wife lives 30 miles away with
two young children with measles?
So in practice, yes.
This duty should not fall to a
pre-registration houseman.
Always make sure that your recipient
of the news is not alone. If he
is, ask him to fetch a friend
into the house. Impress upon
them, where appropriate, the need
to drive safely to the hospital
and not to injure themselves on
the journey.
Always inform the relatives' G.P.
who will need to call.

297. Initially your seniors will help you,
but this is a skill you have to
acquire as a doctor.
Make sure that you are certain of
your facts (e.g. have a written
histology) and that your seniors
have authorised you to speak to
the relatives.
Insist on conducting the interview
in a private room and, if you are
wise, in the presence of a senior
nurse.
There is still something in the
notion of primitive peoples who
kill the bearer of bad tidings so,
when you have said your piece and
done your best, withdraw and allow
the nurse to continue the consoling.

298. How often should the H.S. visit
     all his patients?

299. Has the Operation Consent Form much
     legal validity and any importance?

300. May a 15 year old pregnant girl
     sign a consent form for an
     appendicectomy?

301. In an emergency concerning a child,
     will telephoned verbal consent
     by a parent suffice for an
     operation?

298. Jobs vary, and you should try to
     avoid duplicating your seniors'
     round.
     A full ward round should be done
     by one member of the team every
     day.
     On evenings off, you should go
     quickly round all the patients
     before you leave and mention any
     problems to both the nurse in
     charge <u>and</u> your colleague deputy.
     When on <u>duty</u>, you should go quickly
     round all your patients with the
     night nurse after she has come
     on duty.

299. Not much validity, but it may become
     quite important.
     As a legal document it is incorrectly
     witnessed because the witness
     (the doctor who gives the explan-
     ation) is one of the parties
     involved, and is not independent.
     It may be quite important as
     corroboration for the statement
     that a reasonable attempt was made
     to explain things to the patient.

300. No. Although she may be old enough
     to be given contraceptives without
     parental knowledge, or to
     conceive, she is not old enough to
     sign a consent form until she is
     16 years. Before this her parent
     or guardian must sign.

301. Yes.
     It is wise, where possible, for the
     actual surgeon who will operate
     to obtain this consent, preferably
     in front of a witness.
     He should then complete a Consent
     Form and the witness countersign
     it.

302.   How should waiting relatives be
       informed of a patient's death?

303.   What factors govern when a post-
       operative patient is 'fit' for
       discharge home?

302. There can be no hard and fast rules, but our joint advice is as follows.

Discuss with the senior ward nurse on duty which of you is better placed to inform the relatives. Frequently the nurse will have developed a special rapport with them during terminal illness, and will wish to undertake the duty herself, merely offering them the option of seeing the doctor as well.

Otherwise, insist on the nurse accompanying you; give a suitably expurgated account of the death, and retire. She will offer 'tea and sympathy'.

303. There are three factors:
   i) whether he is 'medically fit' to be discharged.
  ii) whether the home circumstances are suitable.
 iii) whether the G.P.'s team is happy with these arrangements.

Remember that almost nothing is so destructive to a patient's morale as ignominious re-admission to hospital only days after cheerful discharge from the same bed.

Two patients with identical physical illnesses and treatments may be correctly discharged home at completely different times because one has two sons and an unemployed daughter living in the same bungalow, whereas the other lives in a top flat with an invalid husband.

304.   How soon after admission should the
       prudent H.S. start to concern
       himself about the possible future
       arrangements for a patient's
       discharge home?

305.   Young patients who have had
           relatively minor operations can
           be sent home at virtually any
           mutually convenient moment.
       Elderly patients after big operations
           often require a carefully planned
           discharge home.
       Who should be involved, and are there
           any simple guidelines on timing?

304.   Elective cases: immediately,
                        examine the 'social
                        history' with a view
                        to ultimate discharge
                        home.
        Emergency cases:very soon post-
                        operatively.
        A considerable improvement in bed usage
            can be sustained by the simple
            practice of identifying early those
            patients who live alone, have many
            stairs, etc. so that any home
            arrangements can be timed to
            coincide with physical recovery.

305.   Once your chief and your ward sister
            both agree that discharge is
            imminent, you must ring the
            patient's G.P.   He is the lynch-
            pin of all home arrangements as,
            if they crumble, it will be he who
            has to sort out the mess, not you.
        The G.P. and M.S.W.*will arrange for
            the district/practice nurse to
            visit, meals-on-wheels, home
            help etc.
        Timing: Give the G.P. and his team
            adequate warning.
                Send 'problem' patients home
            early rather than late in the day.
                Do not send 'problem' patients
            home at the weekends or on Bank
            Holidays unless the G.P. expressly
            agrees to this.
        Make sure that your patient takes with
            him your handwritten discharge note
            which should state: diagnosis,
                        operation, any compli-
                        cations, treatments on
                        discharge, and your
                        Consultant's and your
                        own name, both written
                        legibly.

        (* M.S.W. = Medical Social Worker.)

Neurosurgery

306.   How urgent is the treatment of a
       suspected cerebral abscess?

307.   Outline the classical presentation
       of an extradural haemorrhage.
       Why is early diagnosis so
       important?

308.   Staff nurse rings you up at 2.00 a.m.
       and tells you that one of your
       patients has fallen out of bed and
       hit his head. What should you do?

306.   The urgency is paramount.
        Correct treatment holds out the
            possibility of a complete cure.
        This diagnostic label will secure
            instant admission to any neuro-
            surgical unit.
        Lumbar puncture to exclude the
            differential diagnosis (meningitis)
            is excessively risky, often fatal,
            and should only be done after
            neurosurgical consultation.

307.   Young person, often a child.
        Sharp blow on temple   K.O'd.
            recovers after a few minutes (the
            'lucid interval'). Look for a
            scalp swelling.
        Slow onset increasing intracerebral
            pressure.
        Headache + local pain.
        Vomiting.
        Drowsiness or irritability, brady-
            cardia, rising B.P.
        Weakness on opposite side of body
            (frequently absent).
        Dilated pupil on the same side of body
            (IIIrd nerve palsy).
        Unconsciousness,
        Death.
        Diagnosis is important because early
            operative decompression will cure
            this potentially fatal injury.

308.   You must get up and see the patient both
            for humanitarian reasons and because
            if you do not, you place yourself in
            an impossible position.
        Ask both the nurse and patient what
            happened.
        Examine the bony skeleton for tender-
            ness and conduct a brief neuro-
            logical examination. This must
            include the base line observations
            of level of consciousness, pulse,
            blood pressure and respiration,
            pupil size, reaction to light.
        It is traditional to order immediate
            skull x-rays if the patient was
            knocked out but the reasoning behind
            this is insecure - they can probably
            wait until next morning.

309.   What is the purpose in taking x-rays
       after a head injury?

310.   Do you admit all head injuries seen
       in Casualty? If not, what
       governs admission policy?

311.   Do you think patients correctly
       sent home from Casualty after
       an apparently minor head injury
       should take any analgesics?

309.   Controversial.
        a) to look for fractures. This is
           particularly important in cases
           of assault, with medico-legal
           implications.
        b) to help the surgeon choose a site
           for his burr hole.
        c) to identify a depressed fracture
           that needs elevation (to avoid
           late epilepsy).
        d) as a factor influencing the timing
           of discharge from hospital.

310.   Controversial.
        It is logistically impossible to
        admit every person seen in
        Casualty with a head injury.
        Thus a selection must be made.
        The question is probably best
        answered the other way round:
        send home only
        a) Those not knocked out.
        b) Those fully conscious without
           neurological signs.
        c) Those without skull fracture (if
           their case has merited x-ray).
        d) Those who have a home to go to
           where they will not be left
           alone for the first 24 hours.
        If there are any doubts, it is safer
        to retain the patient overnight,
        particularly children.

311.   Yes, of course, but only in moderation.
        Instruct the patient that it is quite
        safe for an adult to take one or two
        tablets of paracetemol or aspirin
        4 hourly for headache.
        Avoid alcohol.
        Severe unresponsive headache, vomiting,
           weakness or confusion all require
           immediate review by either G.P. or
           Casualty Department.

312.   Is follow up of patients sent home
        from from Casualty with 'minor'
        head injuries important?
        How should it be done?

313.   Outline the classic presentation
        of a chronic subdural haematoma.

314.   How may subdural haematoma be
        diagnosed?

312.   Yes - slowly developing subdural
        haematoma may take several days
        to become apparent.
        Give a patient a note to the G.P.
        and make it clear that you
        expect the patient to be examined
        by him after two or three days.

313.   The initial head injury may be overt
        or so trivial that it passes
        unnoticed.
        Usually, but not invariably, it
        affects older people.
        Gradual development of drowsiness
        over several days to several
        weeks.
        Personality change $\pm$ incontinence.
        Localising signs (e.g. hemiparesis)
        occur late.
        The diagnosis is often missed until
        later, because of a low index of
        suspicion.
        Some die of this remediable condition,
        wrongly ascribed to 'old age'.

314.   Diagnosis is usually not too difficult,
        once you have considered its
        possibility.
        History and clinical examination may
        suggest the diagnosis.
        Confirm by 1) Skull fracture (often
                       absent).
                   2) Midline shift shown by
                       shift in calcified
                       pineal gland $\pm$ brain
                       scan.
                   3) C.T. scan shows the
                       haematoma.
        Evacuation leads to an improvement,
        dependent on how much irrevocable
        damage has already occurred.

315.   You are asked to see a head injury
        in Casualty with watery fluid
        coming out of an ear. What does
        this mean, and what should you do
        about it?

316.   What should you do with an
        obstreperous, confused head
        injury patient who is disturbing
        the sleep of the rest of the
        ward?

315. This is C.S.F. otorrhoea.
This means that there must be a
fracture of the petrous temporal
bone.
A gentle auroscopic examination is
possible, but usually contributes
little (blood clot obscures).
Do not plug the ear, let the C.S.F.
flow out.
Start prophylactic antibiotics to
prevent meningitis.
Admit the patient to hospital.
These leaks usually stop spontaneously
within a few days.

316. Your principal guide to the progress
of a head injury is the level of
consciousness.
Place him in a side room with
adequate (male) nursing where
possible.
Obtain senior sanction for this, and
use either human or the least
physical restraint necessary
(i.e. use cot restraints, tying
wrists).
You must recognise that any sedation
carries a real risk, thus you may
mask the signs of intracerebral
compression - and end up with a
quiet but dead patient.
Occasionally you just have to use
light sedation, but be sure that
you are doing this to treat your
patient, and not the others in
the ward! Promazine (Sparine)
12.5 - 25 mg is probably the best.

317.   You are called to the Casualty
        Department urgently to see a
        25 year old woman who is lying
        quietly, breathing easily, and
        is unconscious. What should you
        do?

318.   Outline the classic features of
        moderately raised intracranial
        pressure in an adult.

319.   What does a right homonymous
        hemianopia mean?

317.   Confirm that there is a good volume
        pulse of a reasonable rate and
        the airway is clear.
        Turn her semiprone.
        The differential diagnosis is:
        1) Diabetic hypoglycaemia.
        2) Post-epileptic fit.
        3) Overdose of drugs ± alcohol.
        4) Head injury.
        5) Other.
        Exclude diabetic hypoglycaemia by
        inserting a large intravenous
        needle, withdraw blood for
        dextrostix and glucose estimation
        and insert 50 ml of 50% dextrose.
        If the patient wakes up, you have
        the diagnosis - if not, you have
        done no harm.
        Look for signs of an epileptic fit,
        e.g. wet or soiled pants.
        Seek a history from ambulance men etc.
        Conduct a neurological examination.
        remember to look for neck stiffness
        (subarachnoid haemorrhage).
        The size of the pupils may help: large
        with alcohol, small with opiates.
        Do barbiturate levels/drug screen.
        Ponder.

318.   Headache,
        Vomiting,
        Papilloedema.
        In chronically raised I.C.P. a
        lateral skull x-ray will show
        erosion of the pituitary fossa.

319.   The patient loses appreciation of
        his right hand field of view.
        He cannot see the lateral field of
        the right eye, and the medial of
        the left. Thus the lesion must
        be behind the optic chiasma and
        is not peripheral, but central
        (optic tract).

320. Distinguish hemiplegia from
       paraplegia.

321. Distinguish dysphasia from dysarthria.

322. What are the systemic signs of
       acutely rising intracranial
       pressure?

323. In a patient with neurological
       signs of a lumbar disc protrusion,
       how may the tendon jerks indicate
       the level?

320.   Hemiplegia is paralysis of the whole
        of one side of the body (e.g. left).
        Paraplegia is paralysis of both legs
        usually due to spinal cord damage.

321.   Dysphasia may be sensory - patient
        does not comprehend sensory
        input, e.g. "put out your tongue"
        evokes no response.
        or motor - patient appears to
        understand, but articulates
        successfully the wrong words in
        reply, which annoys him.
        Dysarthria - sensori-motor aspects
        of comprehension intact; but the
        words are articulated wrongly,
        e.g. cerebellar scanning speech.

322.   Drowsiness/unconsciousness - level
        of consciousness is the best
        guide.
        Slow pulse)
        High blood) i.e. the exact <u>reverse</u>
        pressure) of haemorrhage.
        Eventually, respiratory irregularity
        e.g. Cheyne Stokes.

323.   Knee jerk reduced - L 3/4.
        Great toe dorsiflexion reduced - L 5.
        Ankle jerks reduced - S 1.

324.   When should damaged peripheral
        nerves be repaired?

325.   A middle aged man develops leg
        weakness, and you elicit a
        history of two months inter-
        scapular back pain.
        What is the most likely cause?
        How urgent is referral?

324. Controversial.
The classical answer is to clean
the wound, mark the nerves, allow
healing and refer for secondary
nerve suture at four weeks.
Simple small nerves, cleanly cut do
well with primary nerve suture
(e.g. digital nerves).
Many surgeons are extending this
concept for the larger nerves
using operating microscopes.
Reports show variable results in
different centres.
Certainly a young person with a major
nerve injury should be given the
benefit of early consultation with
a surgeon skilled in these procedures,
and on some, he will advocate immediate repair.

325. Extradural compression of the spinal
cord by metastatic disease (e.g. Ca.
prostate).
Seek a sensory level.
Penetrated thoracic spine A-P views
are helpful to show collapse or
sclerosis.
This is a neurosurgical emergency:
cord recovery is directly propor-
tional to compression time.
Immediate neurosurgical consultation is
indicated, even at night.

Ophthalmological Surgery

326. A patient presents with a three day
history of sore red eyes, and
lids that are crusted and sticky
in the morning, without impair-
ment of visual acuity.
Give the probable diagnosis and
differential diagnosis.
Outline your treatment.

327. What is the main risk for the inexpert
in prescribing eye drops which
contain steroids?

328. When should you send a patient home
from the Casualty Department
with the eye covered?

326.   <u>Acute Conjunctivitis</u>
        a) Bacterial: the majority
                      visual acuity normal
                      take a culture swab
                      antibiotics, e.g.
                          Chloramphenicol 2-4 hrly
                          & nocte
                      never use steroids
                      personal hygiene is
                          important: the examiner
                          and patient must wash
                          their hands
        b) Viral: less common
                  visual acuity often impaired
                  by corneal inflammation
                  (keratitis)
              or Adenovirus, often epidemic
                  Herpes virus (dendritic ulcer)
                  avoid steroid ointments

327.   If applied to an eye containing Herpes
        simplex virus (dendritic ulcer)
        they cause it to spread causing
        permanent corneal opacity.
        So easy is it for the inexperienced
        to miss the Herpes (e.g. in
        addition to a corneal abrasion)
        that steroid drops are banned in
        many Casualty Departments, and our
        advice is that only specialist
        ophthalmologists should prescribe
        them.

328.   1) If you have anaesthetised the
           protective blink reflex
           (e.g. corneal amethocaine).
        2) If you have dilated one pupil
           (and also paralysed accommo-
           dation on that side).
        3) If you have instilled an opaque
           eye medication, e.g. Chloram-
           phenicol gel, some recommend
           covering the eye, some do not.
        When you have pronounced an eye
           undamaged, do not cover it!

329.   What is the most important single
       observation to record about an
       injured eye?

330.   A mother has been poked in the eye
       by her baby and presents with a
       painful photophobic eye (photo-
       phobia is pain in the eye when
       exposed to light caused by
       ciliary muscle spasm).
       How should you examine her?
       What is the probable diagnosis?

331.   How would you treat a patient with a
       simple recent corneal abrasion?

329.   Visual acuity.
       It sounds so obvious, doesn't it,
          that you <u>must</u> discover whether
          the patient can see out of the
          eye; but this information is
          very often lacking.
       It is more important that the patient
          can see out, than that you can
          see in!
       If the patient wears spectacles,
          make sure that he puts them on
          first ('corrected' visual acuity)
          or, if not, test vision through
          a 2 mm pinhole in a piece of
          card held close to the eye.
       Apart from its clinical significance
          a record of visual acuity may
          have important medico-legal
          implications.

330.   The pain may be so severe that it
          precludes an adequate view. If
          so, instil a few drops of local
          anaesthetic, e.g. amethocaine.
       Use fluorescein (wash away any
          excess) to delineate the extent
          of any area of corneal epithelial
          loss, i.e. corneal abrasion.
       Examine under the lids for foreign
          bodies.
       Record visual acuity.
       Examine the depths of the eye with
          an ophthalmoscope or slit-lamp
          (better).
       The probable diagnosis is a simple
          corneal abrasion.

331.   Topical antibiotic e.g. Chloramphenicol
          drops.
       Homatropine drops to dilate the pupil
          and relieve pain from ciliary
          muscle spasm.
       Eye pad.
       Review again next day.
       Any abrasion which fails to respond
          to treatment in 48 hours should
          be referred to the Eye Department.

332.   While using a hammer and chisel,
       a man was aware of a sudden
       sharp discomfort in the eye,
       but thought no more about it
       until the following day when
       he woke with a painful red eye.
    How would you manage this situation?

333.   How do you manage a patient with a
       feeling of a piece of grit under
       the lid?
    Do you need to follow up such
       patients?

332. Take a detailed history and, if
      possible, examine the instrument used.
      Record the best (corrected) visual
      acuity for each eye, testing the
      injured one first.
      Examine the lids and fluorescein-
      stained conjunctiva with a good
      (oblique) light for puncture wounds
      and abrasions.
      Check the pupils for size, equality and
      distortion (a perforating wound may
      be sealed by the iris).
      X-ray the orbit for foreign bodies.
      Examine the depths of the eye with an
      ophthalmoscope or slit-lamp (better).
      Do not palpate the globe for intra-
      ocular pressure.
      Most Eye Departments are anxious to see
      all patients with a history of
      hammer and chisel injury immediately.
      If this is not practicable manage-
      ment depends now on your diagnosis:
      a) Simple corneal abrasion:
         Chloramphenicol, Homatropine, pad.
         See next day.
      b) Corneal foreign body:
         Remove, Chloramphenicol, Homatropine,
         pad. Eye Department 1-2/7.
      c) No diagnosis:
         Refer to Eye Department directly.

333. Record visual acuity.
      Examine the fluorescein-stained cornea
      with an oblique light for an
      associated abrasion (common).
      Evert the lids. A foreign body is
      usually easily seen, and can be
      stroked out with a cotton bud.
      Chloramphenicol ointment. Eye pad.
      A simple subtarsal F.B. needs no
      follow up.
      A subtarsal F.B. + corneal abrasion
      needs follow up for the abrasion
      at 48 hours.

334.   What is a stye?
       How should it be treated?

335.   A welder comes to Casualty complaining
       of 'arc' eye. What is this
       condition, and how would you treat
       it?

336.   A shop-keeper has been attacked and
       a chemical thrown in his face and
       eyes: what is the immediate
       management?

334.   An infection of a lash follicle
        producing a local collection
        of pus and inflammation.
        Hot spoon bathing 4-6 hrly.
        Topical antibiotics q.d.s., e.g.
            Chloramphenicol.
        Occasionally, systemic antibiotics
        for spreading cellulitis.

335.   'Arc' eye is due to acute corneal
        epithelial oedema caused by
        exposure to the welder's arc
        producing severe pain and
        blurred vision, usually some
        hours after the event.
        The initial treatment is dilation
        of the pupil which should be
        maintained with homatropine 2%
        and a topical antibiotic
        (Chloramphenicol); pad the worse
        eye.
        If the pain is severe and vision
        markedly impaired, admission
        should be advised.

336.   Irrespective of the chemical, the
        eye requires copious irrigation,
        ideally with a buffered solution,
        but if none is available, tap
        water will do. If necessary,
        instillation of amethocaine drops
        may facilitate the procedure.
        Particulate matter must be carefully
        sought and removed from the
        conjunctival fornices.
        Urgent ophthalmic care is mandatory.
        Alkali burns of the cornea are much
        more destructive than similar
        acid ones because alkalis can
        penetrate rapidly with deceptively
        less pain.

337.   You are asked to see an agitated,
       tearful 9 year old boy who says
       that he has hurt his eye on a
       twig.
       On examination the eye is bloodshot
       and you have difficulty visualising
       the retina.
       What should you do?

338.   Is subconjunctival haemorrhage a
       serious condition?

337.   The first problem is to examine the
        eye. The child may well keep the
        lids tightly closed. After gentle
        reassurance, lay the child on a
        bed with his head on a pillow; he
        will not then jerk his head back
        from your examining fingers.
        Check the lids for lacerations and
        look under them as he moves the
        eye.
        Record visual acuity if possible,
        pupil sizes and response to light.
        Try to examine the retina.
        Always <u>x-ray</u> the orbit for foreign
        bodies; sometimes you will find
        an air rifle pellet lodged there.
        Use fluorescein to check for corneal
        abrasions.
        Lack of patient co-operation means
        that you now need expert help to
        examine the depths of the eye
        properly; in a tearful child this
        often requires sedation + local,
        or even general anaesthesia.

338.   a) <u>Spontaneous</u>: due to rupture of a
           small blood vessel:- trivial.
           Resolves in three weeks without
           treatment.
        b) <u>Traumatic</u>: usually unimportant.
           But if you cannot see its
           posterior edge, it may indicate
           a basal fracture of the skull.

339.   A 60 year old lady presents with a
       three month's history of inter-
       mittent blurring of vision of
       one eye associated with a mild
       frontal headache, and a one day
       history of more severe orbital
       pain, impaired vision and nausea.
   On examination the eye's visual
       acuity is diminished, the con-
       junctival and episcleral blood
       vessels adjacent to the cornea
       are markedly congested, and the
       cornea looks hazy with an oval
       pupil.

   a) What is the probable diagnosis?
   b) What is the differential diagnosis?
   c) Is it important to secure the
      correct diagnosis?

340.   Cataract is a common cause of
       impaired vision. List seven
       causes.

339. a) Acute glaucoma.
      b) Acute iritis.
      c) Yes, because the treatment of each
         is different and in both cases,
         urgent.
      Expert examination by a slit-lamp is
         necessary to differentiate (a) from
         (b), so immediate referral to the
         Eye Department is required.
      Acute Glaucoma
      Raised intraocular pressure that may
         lead to blindness.
      Due to obstruction of the outflow of
         aqueous humour from the anterior
         chamber because the peripheral
         iris has blocked the trabecular
         meshwork.
      The principal abnormality is a narrow
         angle between iris and cornea.
      Gentle palpation of the globe reveals
         raised intraocular pressure.
      (Chronic glaucoma is caused by
         obstruction beyond the trabecular
         network and presents insidiously
         as a deeply cupped optic disc with
         visual field defects in a hard eye.)

340. Idiopathic associated with ageing
         (common).
      Diabetes mellitus.
      Prolonged treatment with steroids.
      Atopic dermatitis.
      Dystrophia myotonica.
      Congenital.
      Galactosaemia.

341.   A young man has been punched in the
       eye with a fist and the following
       day complains of bruised lids,
       slightly blurred vision, and mild
       diplopia.
       What are the essential steps in your
       management?

342.   a) Is the pupil large or small in
          Horner's syndrome?
       b) What are the other features?
       c) Name one simple investigation
          you could do in such a case?

341.   Record (corrected) visual acuity.
        Check the pupillary reflexes.
        Record eye movements in all directions
            of gaze: bruising or entrapment of
            nerves or muscles may restrict
            ocular movements.
        Test sensation over the cheek (a
            fractured orbital floor may
            damage the intraorbital nerve).
        Examine the globe and its contents.
        X-ray skull and obtain orbital views.

        You should refer this case to the Eye
            Department because you have
            discovered that the injured eye
            malfunctions (blurring and
            diplopia). Remember that blunt
            injury may cause damage to the
            posterior globe ranging from
            retinal oedema to scleral rupture
            despite there being little to be
            seen by the inexperienced from in
            front.

342.   a) Small (but reacts normally to
            light and accommodation).
            (The action of the sympathetic
            is to dilate the pupil e.g. in
            fear).
        b) Mild ptosis, enophthalmos,
            decreased sweating, conjunctival
            hyperaemia.
        c) Chest x-ray: an apical lung lesion
            can pick off the cervical
            sympathetic chain close to its
            origin at T 1.

343.   A metal grinder presents in Casualty
        with a sore red eye, which he
        tells you is due to "swarf".
        What is "swarf"?
        Outline your management.

343.   Swarf is the fine metallic powder
         obtained when metal is ground.
         Swarf in the eye is a very common
            industrial mishap and occurs
            when workmen grind without
            wearing goggles.
         If they present immediately, the
            swarf is visible as tiny black
            particles embedded in the cornea.
         Often the patient waits until the
            next day, and may merely think
            that he has a 'sore eye'. Careful
            inspection will show a slightly
            red sclera and the same small
            black specks now surrounded by a
            ring of dark stain.
         In either case:
         1) Record corrected visual acuity
              carefully: accident claims
              often arise in these cases.
         2) X-ray to exclude penetrating
              metallic injury.
         3) Dislodge superficial F.B. with a
              needle and L.A. Gutt. Homatropine
              2% will ease the discomfort of the
              attendant ciliary spasm, and
              Gutt. Chloramphenicol 0.5% and
              pad is the initial treatment, and
              the patient should be reviewed
              next day.
          4) Refer more complex cases to the Eye
              Department directly.

Orthopaedic Surgery

344. How should you describe a fracture
     if asked to comment on its x-ray?

345. Why may fractured calcaneus often
     be mistreated?

346. What is the usual mechanism of injury
     that causes tearing of a meniscus
     (cartilage) of the knee?

347. Outline the clinical features of
     slipped upper femoral epiphyses.
     Why is early diagnosis important?

344.   Ask for contemporaneous views in
        two different planes at 90° (to
        check displacement).
        Make sure your film includes the
        joints above and below the
        fracture.
        If it is a difficult area (e.g. elbow)
        ask for x-ray of the other (normal)
        side (to check the epiphyses).
        The correct answer must include
        situation, line of fracture,
        displacement, involvement of
        neighbouring joint, soft tissue
        damage, any foreign bodies.

345.   The fracture is often missed. This
        is because although there is
        great local tenderness of the
        heel, there is often no bony
        displacement. Thus it may
        appear to be 'merely a bruise'.
        Always x-ray these heels. If the
        patient cannot stand, admit him
        overnight.
        The associated lumbar vertebral
        crush fracture or pelvic fracture
        may also be missed.

346.   A fall, while both twisting and
        bearing full weight on the bent
        knee. This is why it is a
        common football injury.

347.   It typically occurs in peri-pubertal,
        overweight boys.
        The child develops a slight limp,
        which he often tries to hide and
        belittles to avoid ridicule.
        In early cases it is important to
        identify the only physical sign,
        which is pain on medial rotation
        of the hip.
        X-ray all these cases. Compare both
        sides, the changes are subtle, and
        beware a bilateral slip!
        Early treatment carries a good prognosis.
        Late diagnosis may lead to early
        degenerative changes in the hip and
        to a permanent limp.

348.   What are the basic steps of a Keller's
          operation for bunions?
       Are the results good or bad?

349.   How soon should strapping and
          stretching of a talipes (club)
          foot begin after birth?

350.   What position does the leg assume
          below a fractured neck of femur?
       Does it differ from a patient who
          has a stroke (C.V.A.).

351.   What is the correct order of x-ray
          investigation of a possible
          cervical spine injury?

352.   What are the signs of established
          non-union of a fracture?

348.   Excision of the base of the proximal
        phalanx of the big toe (treats
        the hallux valgus) with trimming
        of the prominent part of the head
        of the first metatarsal (the
        bunion is the bursa), creating a
        fibrous, painless, pseudoarthrosis.
        The convalescence is very painful
        but the long term results are
        excellent.

349.   Immediately. The talipes should be
        noticed at the initial check of
        the baby and treatment commenced.
        The 'next convenient out-patient
        clinic' is far too late.

350.   Yes.
        Fractured neck of femur: leg abducted,
        shortened, externally rotated.
        C.V.A: leg adducted and medially
        rotated.
        (but note that a posterior dislocation
        of the hip looks similar).

351.   Keep the patient still on his stretcher/
        trolley with the neck protected by
        a sand bag.
        Do not leave him unattended.
        a) Plain AP and lateral views, and
        try to include C 7 (technically
        difficult).
        b) Open mouth views of odontoid peg.
        c) Now consult your seniors. If a)
        and b) O.K., proceed to
        d) Views in flexion and extension
        with a doctor holding the head.

352.   Possible deformity, increasing if not
        splinted.
        The fracture can be moved without
        tenderness (just as if the patient
        were anaesthetised).
        Fracture persists on x-ray with
        inadequate or absent callus.

353. Classify by age the typical bony
      injury caused by a fall on the
      outstretched hand.

354. How do you diagnose a fractured
      scaphoid?   Does early diagnosis
      matter?

353.   Less than 5 years - very rare.
        5 - 12 years - greenstick fracture
                        midshaft radius and
                        ulna.
        13 - 17 years - fracture distal radial
                        epiphysis.
        18 - 40 years - fractured scaphoid.
        40 - 55 years - fractured neck of
                        humerus.
        More than 56 years - Colles' fracture.

354.   This fracture is frequently missed
            because the wrist is not examined
            rigorously, and the x-ray signs
            are subtle.
        Clinical signs - slight swelling and
            definite tenderness in the anatomi-
            cal snuff box. You must know
            exactly where to press, and the
            patient will wince.
                        - scaphoid tenderness
            on pinching together thumb and
            and middle finger.
        X-ray   - hairline crack may be
            visible with a magnifying glass.
        Early diagnosis is important. Failure
            to immobilise may result in avascu-
            lar necrosis of the proximal segment
            of the scaphoid bone, leading to
            disabling early secondary arthritis
            of the wrist.
        If in doubt, seek senior advice.
            In general, the wrist is immobilised
            because of the physical signs; and
            P.O.P. treatment is only abandoned
            after several weeks when serial
            x-rays then fail to show any
            fracture.

355.   What important tests should you make
        in a patient with a knife cut
        over the middle phalanx of the
        finger.
        Do these tests influence management?

356.   A G.P. rings you up at night
        wondering whether he should send
        up a man with a painful, slightly
        infected hand, or wait until
        morning. What do you advise?

357.   Would you regard as adequate an
        x-ray that showed a displaced
        fracture of the ulna above a
        normal wrist joint?

355.   a) Tendon function - immobilise wrist
          and metacarpals before testing
          phalangeal movement.
       b) Skin sensation to pin prick - test
          the integrity of the digital
          nerves.

       a) is better retested after you have
          injected local anaesthetic:
          b) cannot be tested then! So,
          first test distally for pin
          prick, then inject anaesthetic,
          and then test the tendons again.
          Tendon repairs require an
          experienced surgeon. Digital
          nerve repair should be done
          primarily and is not really
          within the competence of a
          casualty officer. Ideally it
          should be done by an experienced
          microsurgeon using his microscope.

356.   All painful, potentially septic hands
          need to be seen at once by an
          experienced surgeon. So, you
          should ask him to send the patient
          up directly.
       The golden rule is that pain in the
          hand that prevents the patient
          sleeping requires immediate
          surgical decompression.

357.   No.
       Always x-ray the joints above and
          below any fracture.
       In this case there has to be either
          another fracture (radius or ulna)
          or an elbow dislocation to explain
          the displacement of the radial
          fracture.
       Monteggia fracture - fractured distal
          ulna + dislocated (prox) head of
          radius.

358.   What is a "split plaster"? When are
        they used?

359.   It often happens that you have a
        patient in your ward after an
        R.T.A. with abdominal pain and
        a limb in a plaster cast. What
        should you do if he complains
        of severe pain under the plaster
        and/or in the foot?

358.   The purpose of a plaster of Paris
        splint is to maintain reduction
        of a fracture.
        Over the first 24 hours the soft
        tissues tend to swell with
        haematoma, and if the limb is
        enclosed in a rigid plaster
        shell, internal pressure increases
        and the blood vessels may be
        occluded leading to distal gangrene.
        To avoid this sequence, the limb is
        padded inside the plaster which
        is then split with a knife from
        end to end and the padding cut
        with scissors down to the skin -
        thus allowing some expansion of
        the limb.
        After a week or so, the haematoma
        will start to absorb. The limb
        will shrink again, and the P.O.P.
        become loose. It will then need
        reinforcement or "completion",
        or replacement.

359.   You must not ignore this information.
        Adequately immobilised fractures
        are not tremendously painful.
        Go and examine the limb in a good
        light.
        If there is any doubt about the
        distal circulation, the plaster
        must be split wider. In severe
        cases, it may need to be removed
        and traction instituted.
        If the pain is under the P.O.P., this
        may indicate local pressure and a
        window may be cut over it.
        In all cases you need to inform both
        your own Registrar and the ortho-
        paedic surgeon who applied the
        plaster at once: it will not wait
        until morning. You should also
        record your findings in the case
        notes.

360.   You are standing in for the ortho-
       paedic H.S., and you are asked
       to see a 6 year old child in
       their ward who last night had a
       supracondylar fracture of the
       humerus reduced and is now
       complaining of pain in the hand.
       What tests should you do?

361.   Do you think that a young man with
       a fractured shaft of femur will
       require a blood transfusion?

362.   Distinguish between an osteo-
       arthritic and a rheumatoid
       hand.

360.   The danger of a supracondylar fracture
        of the humerus is that the bony
        fragment may compress the brachial
        artery, leading to distal ischaemia,
        or soft tissue swelling may compress
        its branches in the forearm.
        Feel the hand for warmth.
        Feel the radial pulse and compare it
        with that of the other wrist:
        however remember that a palpable
        pulse is still compatible with
        forearm ischaemia.
        Pain on gentle passive extension of
        the fingers and wrist is an early
        indication of forearm ischaemia,
        and must not be ignored.
        Do not alter the position of the arm
        yourself but record your findings
        in the case notes, and inform the
        responsible Orthopaedic Registrar
        or Consultant - immediately.

361.   Yes - usually.
        The perforating branches of the
        profunda femoris artery are
        certain to have been torn and an
        adult thigh will accommodate at
        least 1.5 litres of haematoma
        without even appearing to be
        tremendously swollen.
        You should reckon that the fracture
        will need two units of blood.

362.   Osteoarthritis - affects wrist,
        thumb MCP joint, distal I-P
        joints (Heberden's nodes).
        Rheumatoid - affects wrist, MCP
        joints, thumb and tendons of
        fingers.
        There are about ten recognised
        deformities!

363.   How do you distinguish a bad sprain
       from a fractured ankle? Does
       this distinction matter?

364.   Supracondylar fracture of the
       humerus is not a particularly
       common injury: so why do you
       need to know about it?
       In whom does it occur?
       Who should reduce it?

363.   a) Careful palpation will usually
          reveal whether the tenderness
          is actually over the bony
          malleoli (fracture), or over
          the ligaments just distally
          (sprain).
       b) Abnormal movement of the ankle
          secondary to ligament rupture
          may require E.U.A.to confirm
          the diagnosis.
       c) The distinction may be important
          medico-legally, but often not
          clinically: an undisplaced
          hairline fracture can be
          managed in the same way as a
          bad sprain. A displaced fracture
          needs expert management.
       d) Sprains are best treated sympto-
          matically with early physio-
          therapy to reduce swelling,
          regain mobility and re-educate
          damaged proprioceptive mechanisms.
       e) Fractures should be seen by an
          orthopaedic surgeon and some
          require operative fixation.

364.   The main risk with this essentially
       'ordinary' fracture is the com-
       plication of brachial artery
       occlusion with permanent ischaemic
       damage to the child's forearm and
       hand.
       Supracondylar fracture of the humerus
       occurs in children (4 - 10 years)
       who fall on their arms.
       The distal humerus and forearm are
       displaced backwards and upwards
       (triceps spasm). This causes the
       brachial vessels to be bowstrung
       over the sharp, anteriorly displaced
       proximal fragment.
       Check the radial pulse and integrity of
       radial, median and ulnar nerves.
       Never attempt to reduce this fracture
       yourself. You may damage the
       artery you are trying to preserve.
       This reduction must be done by an
       experienced orthopaedic surgeon
       under full relaxation analgesia.

365.   Outline your pre-operative management
       of an otherwise fit 75 year old
       lady who arrives in Casualty with
       a displaced fractured neck of femur.

366.   What types of crystal are known to
       be associated with arthropathy?

367.   If you had to sustain an uncomplicated
       leg fracture, which would you
       prefer - shaft of femur, upper
       tibia and fibula, or lower tibia
       + fibula?

365. 1) Diagnosis - this is obvious, the
leg is shortened, externally
rotated and the hip tender.
2) Analgesia - give small doses of
IV opiates (e.g. Pethidine
10-15 mg) + antiemetic
(Perphenazine 5 mg IV).
3) X-ray - chest (pre-op) and hip,
PA and lateral.
4) Traction - set up skin traction
to the foot. 5-6 lb. straight
pull, ventifoam is adequate.
Cover this manoeuvre with more
IV Pethidine - once traction is
set up, the pain is much reduced.
5) Settle the patient in the ward.
Reassess analgesia requirements.
Clerk her and arrange urgent elective
operation. Remember that it is
disgraceful cruelty to manipulate
or transport a patient with an
obvious fracture without first
giving analgesia.

366. Urate (gout).
Calcium pyrophosphate (pseudo-gout,
chondrocalcinosis and possibly
primary osteoarthritis).
Hydroxyapatite.

367. Fractured shaft of femur. These are
relatively easy to align and heal
well.
Upper tibia and fibula is a rarer
injury, and more difficult to align
but they unite adequately.
Lower third tibia + fibula has a justly
awful reputation for mal-union and
non-union. Although things may go
well for you, you may face months,
years or even permanent disability
after this fracture.

368. What principles govern the diagnosis and management of a fractured patella?

369. Classify hand infections by anatomical site.

370. Why are incisions on the dorsum of an infected hand seldom indicated?

368.   In a young person x-ray the other
        side - your 'fracture' may be
        the midline epiphysis!
        The key observation is whether the
        'extensor mechanism' (quadriceps
        muscle, tendon, patella, ligaments,
        tibial tubercle) has been dis-
        rupted, or not: i.e. can the
        patient straighten his knee?
        a) extensor mechanism intact: this is
           the relatively trivial injury of
           cracked patella.
           Aspirate any knee haematoma.
           Apply P.O.P. cylinder only.
        b) ruptured extensor mechanism:
           immediate operation to repair
           the quadriceps tendon ± fixation
           of the patella or patellectomy.
        c) follow up of all patellar injuries
           is needed as a rough posterior
           surface may lead to knee joint
           damage and require later
           elective patellectomy.

369.   a) Terminal pulp space) these represent
           infection.   ) 90% of acute
        b) Paronychia.   ) localised hand
) infections
        c) Subcutaneous infection.
        d) Palm and web space infection.
        e) Tendon sheath infection.
        f) Infective arthritis.

370.   Infections localised to the dorsum of
        the hand are usually boils or
        carbuncles which do not need
        incision. Dorsal swelling is more
        commonly due to palmar infection
        which may need a palmar incision.

371.   You see an elderly lady in Casualty
        who has fallen and sustained a
        V-shaped deep cut over her lower
        shin. Is this a common injury?
        How would you treat it?

371.   Yes, regrettably very common.
This is a notorious site for poor
    healing. The blood supply of
    the skin here is bad anyway,
    and the apex of the 'V' will
    probably die whatever you do.
    Any haematoma will stretch the
    skin even tighter and cause
    widespread necrosis. Tight
    primary suture is to be avoided.
Recognise that this is not a trivial
    injury.
Clean the wound; if there are no
    gaping raw areas, steristrip it
    and bandage firmly from toes to
    knee and encourage mobilisation.
    Usually there is an area which
    cannot be closed, or closed only
    with tension; cover it with one
    layer of paraffin gauze, and
    then apply a viscopaste or
    similar bandage from the toes to
    just below the knee. Mobilise
    immediately and encourage patient
    to continue walking. Change the
    bandage weekly or fortnightly
    depending on the amount of fluid
    discharge. Debride the wound at
    each dressing change. This avoids
    admission to hospital, reduces the
    risk of D.V.T. and the wound always
    heals eventually.

372. Congenital dislocation of the hip
      and dislocatable hip have been
      described as probably the most
      important asymptomatic congenital
      abnormalities to detect. Why is
      this, and what should be done,
      how and when?

373. Discuss the principles underlying
      both conservative and operative
      management of osteoarthritis of
      the hip?

372. It is important because
   a) It is common: about 1% of neonates
      have a hip abnormality in the
      first two days of life, girls
      commoner than boys.
   b) Early detection and treatment is
      usually simple and effective.
   c) Late detection makes treatment
      more difficult, and often results
      in permanent damage, surgery on
      adolescents or adults, and later
      problems with childbirth.

   All neonatal hips should be examined
   12-36 hours using Barlow's
   manoeuvre. A positive test is
   indicated by a 'clunk' or jerk
   (not a click) as the femoral head
   snaps back into its socket. All
   positive cases should be referred
   immediately to either an orthopaedic or a paediatric firm,
   depending on hospital policy.

   Treatment ranges from merely the
   wearing of two nappies to full
   immobilisation in an abduction
   splint.

373. a) Conservative: simple measures such
      as heel raise, walking stick,
      analgesics, physiotherapy.
   b) Surgical: (i) Manipulation under
                    anaesthesia may
                    be of benefit.
              (ii) Femoral osteotomy -
                    realignment of
                    worn joint surfaces.
             (iii) Arthroplasty -
                    commonest type is
                    total hip replace-
                    ment.
              (iv) Arthrodesis -
                    occasionally used
                    in younger patients.

374.   List the complications of total
         hip replacement.

374.
    (i) Those of any operation -
        anaesthetic, chest,
        D.V.T. etc.

   (ii) Infection - may be early or
        late and may be disastrous
        when cement has been used.
        The prosthesis may need to
        be removed to secure
        healing resulting in a dead
        space forming a pseud-
        arthrosis with gross
        shortening of the leg.

  (iii) Loosening - causing pain.

   (iv) Fracture of the prosthesis
        itself.

    (v) Para-articular ossification
        (of the soft tissues around
        the hip joint).

Paediatric Surgery

375.   What type of inguinal hernia occurs
in children? What is the correct
management?

376.   What is the danger of an inguinal
hernia in infancy and how is it
managed?

377.   What is the commonest hernia in
infancy?
What is the usual history?

378.   What is exomphalos?

379.   What is an epigastric hernia?

380.   What is phimosis?

375.   Indirect.
        Surgical repair - there is no place
        for a truss.

376.   Irreducibility leading to strangu-
        lation. Therefore they should
        be repaired as soon as possible.
        If strangulation occurs, the hernia
        must be reduced within 6 hours,
        otherwise infarction may occur.
        After reduction, the hernia must
        be repaired within a few days to
        prevent recurrence.

377.   True umbilical hernia.* Most resolve
        by one year of age or in the next
        few years.
        Repair is essentially for cosmetic
        reasons and may be carried out
        before the child goes to school
        if requested.

        *Infants have true umbilical hernias,
        adults develop paraumbilical ones.

378.   A congenital defect of the abdominal
        wall at the umbilicus. Abdominal
        viscera prolapse into a hemi-
        spherical opalescent sac at the
        base of the umbilical cord. The
        patient must be transferred to a
        surgical unit. The best dressing
        of the lesion is a sterile sheet
        of polythene.

379.   A hernia of extraperitoneal fat
        through a small midline supra-
        umbilical defect in the linea
        alba. Surgery is indicated if
        it causes pain.

380.   An acquired scar of the foreskin
        causing narrowing of its meatus,
        usually presenting about 8-10 years
        old. (Adults more often develop
        paraphimosis.)

381.   What are the indications for
            circumcision in a child?

382.   What are the contraindications to
            circumcision in a child?

383.   What are the three chief features
            of hypospadias?

384.   Are hydroceles in children usually
            communicating or non-communicating?
        What usually happens in infants'
            hydroceles?

385.   What serious pathology may mimic
            a hydrocele in children?

386.   What is the main differential
            diagnosis of undescended testis?

381. a) True cicatrising phimosis - not
         just a non-retractable fore-
         skin without scars.
      b) Recurrent balanitis (relative
         indication).
      c) Paraphimosis (relative indication
         before puberty).

382. a) Hypospadias.
      b) Medical conditions e.g. haemophilia.
      c) Ammoniacal dermatitis - commonly
         only present as a 'sore foreskin'.

383. a) Proximally placed ventral meatus,
         sometimes stenosed.
      b) Hooded foreskin.
      c) Chordee (not always present).

384. Communicating - i.e. there is a
      patent processus vaginalis.
      Most resolve by one year old.

385. Testicular tumour. Rare, malignant
      usually, but curable by surgery
      if treated early.

386. Retractile testis. The best age to
      differentiate is in the first
      year of life.

387.   What are the indications for
       orchidopexy (the surgical
       correction of undescended
       testicle)?

388.   At what age should a boy with
       cryptorchidism be referred
       to a surgeon?

389.   A child presents with a history
       of acute scrotal pain. What
       is the likely diagnosis? Is
       treatment urgent?

390.   What are the other causes of an
       "acute scrotum"?

391.   What is the natural history of a
       "strawberry naevus"?

387.   There is no single absolute indi-
         cation, but the following points
         should be considered:
         a) Temperature - spermatogenesis is
            less efficient at the higher
            temperature of the abdomen.
         b) Tumour - maldescent is associated
            with an increase risk of x10-30.
            If this occurs it is easier to
            detect if testis has been placed
            in the scrotum.
         c) Torsion - more likely in cryp-
            torchid testis until fixed.
         d) Trauma - said to be more likely
            to an inguinal testis.
         e) "Social and psychological".

388.   As soon as the diagnosis is suspected.
         A few testes may descend in the
         first year of life, but there is
         evidence that pathological changes
         occur before 2 years of age in
         those left inside the abdomen.

389.   Torsion of testis. Epididymitis is
         very rare in children.
         Operation should be performed within
         the hour of hospital admission if
         these ischaemic testicles are to
         be saved.

390.   a) Torsion of appendix testis.
         b) Idiopathic scrotal oedema.
         c) Orchitis e.g. mumps (rare).

391.   It is not present at birth, but
         appears around 3 weeks of age
         and grows for a few months. It
         then begins to resolve after
         2 or 3 years, commencing with
         pallor at the centre.

392.   A babe is born to a mother who
       suffered from hydramnios and
       is noted to be "mucousy" at
       birth.   What is the likely
       diagnosis? What is the immedi-
       ate management?

393.   What is the classical x-ray sign
       of duodenal atresia and how
       does the condition present?

394.   Meconium ileus is a neonatal mani-
       festation of what systemic
       disease?

395.   What, briefly, is Hirschsprung's
       disease?

396.   What are the main two groups of
       anorectal anomaly (imperforate
       anus)?

392.   Oesophageal atresia and tracheo-
       oesophageal fistula. The babe
       should not be fed (sometimes
       the diagnosis is not made until
       the first feed) but the diagnosis
       confirmed by passing a size 10 f.g.
       radio-opaque nasogastric tube,
       which is stopped 10 cm from the
       lips. The babe is transferred to
       a neonatal surgical unit, head up
       15° and keeping the blind upper
       pouch sucked out.

393.   "Double bubble trouble", i.e. two
       air-fluid levels in the upper
       abdomen on the erect film. They
       present with bile-stained vomiting
       in the first 24 hours of life with
       a scaphoid abdomen. 10% of these
       patients are mongols (Down's
       syndrome).

394.   Fibrocystic disease = cystic fibrosis =
       mucoviscidosis. The clinical
       presentation is delayed passage of
       meconium, abdominal distension and
       vomiting.

395.   Absence of ganglion cells in the bowel
       wall, extending proximally for a
       variable distance from the anus.
       It presents with delayed passage
       of meconium (often explosive
       deflation after P.R.), abdominal
       distension and vomiting; male
       preponderance of 4:1.

396.   a) High or supralevator where the
          rectum ends above the pelvic
          floor, usually with a fistula
          to vagina, or in boys, urethra.
       b) Low or infralevator. Usually
          there is a cutaneous fistula.

397.   On which side does a diaphragmatic
       hernia usually occur?   Describe
       the main clinical features.

398.   What antenatal screening test can
       detect most cases of neural
       tube defect?

399.   A child with a C.S.F. shunt for
       hydrocephalus is unwell. What
       must be suspected?

400.   A child of 9 months develops colicky
       abdominal pain, goes pale and
       draws his knees up with the pain.
       What is the likely diagnosis?
       What common signs may be present
       and how is it managed?

401.   Why is appendicitis of special
       importance in children under
       5 years?

397.   Left.   They commonly present as
       neonatal respiratory distress.
       The apex beat is displaced to
       the right and bowel sounds may
       be heard in the chest.   The
       abdomen is flat.   A nasogastric
       tube is passed to reduce intes-
       tinal gas and the patient
       intubated and ventilated, if
       necessary, before transfer to a
       surgical unit.

398.   Serum alpha-foetoprotein level.
       Confirmation is derived from
       the amniotic concentration and by
       ultrasound.

399.   Shunt blockage until disproved.
       This may be manifest in many
       ways, ranging from non-specific
       symptoms to vomiting, headache,
       drowsiness and coma.

400.   Intussusception.   "Red currant
       jelly stool" and an abdominal
       mass.   If fit enough, hydro-
       static reduction by barium
       enema under screening super-
       vision, otherwise laparotomy.

401.   There is frequently a delay in
       presentation and usually
       perforation has occurred before
       diagnosis.   This leads to severe
       fluid imbalance, so resuscitation
       and preoperative antibiotics are
       necessary.

402. An 8 year old presents with diffuse
     abdominal pain, flushed, ill-
     looking, with a fever of 39.5^{0}.
     Is appendicitis likely and what
     other diagnoses should you
     consider?

403. A 9 year old child is admitted with
     2 weeks' malaise and a few days'
     abdominal pain. There is a fever,
     possibly mild hypertension, diffuse
     abdominal tenderness and a
     petechial rash over the buttocks
     and legs. The urine contains
     protein and blood. What is the
     diagnosis?

404. What is the most likely cause of
     major rectal bleeding in a 3 year
     old?

405. What are the commonest causes of
     gastro-intestinal haemorrhage in
     children?

406. What are the three cardinal signs
     of pyloric stenosis?

407. What is the proper management of
     pyloric stenosis?

408. What common cystic lesion is found
     at the lateral end of the eye
     brow?

402.   Appendicitis is unlikely unless there
        is diffuse peritonitis. These
        cases are difficult to evaluate,
        but think of:
        a) Viral infections - usually non-
           specific, but occasionally
           measles etc.
        b) Otitis media or tonsillitis.
        c) Pneumonia.
        d) Pyelonephritis.
        e) Glandular fever.

403.   Henoch-Schönlein purpura.
        This is probably an autoimmune disease
           following a *Strep*. sore throat. It
           is self-limiting and managed
           medically, though visceral compli-
           cations may sometimes call for
           surgery.

404.   Meckel's diverticulum.

405.   a) Neonates - volvulus, fissure in
           ano, acute ulcer.
        b) Infants - fissure, intussusception.
        c) 6 months to 3 years - intussusception,
           Meckel's diverticulum.
        d) Over 3 years - polyps, fissures.

406.   Projectile vomiting, visible peri-
        stalsis, palpable pyloric tumour.

407.   a) Correct any dehydration and hypo-
           chloraemic alkalosis, then
        b) Ramstedt's pyloromyotomy.

408.   External angular dermoid.

409.   What is the likely differential
       diagnosis of a midline cystic
       swelling of the neck?

410.   A child has a soft cystic swelling
       in the side of the neck -
     a) What is the likely diagnosis and
        what single test will support
        this?
     b) What complications occur not
        infrequently?

411.   What are the two commonest causes
       of death in children in the
       U.K.?

412.   What is the commonest solid abdomi-
       nal malignancy in childhood, and
       how does it present?

413.   What are the commonest abnormalities
       of the urinary tract in children?

409.   a) Thyroglossal cyst - excision
           should be carried out before
           it becomes inflamed, because
           after inflammation there is
           a greater risk of recurrence.
        b) Midline dermoid.
        c) Lymph node.

410.   a) Cystic hygroma. They freely
           transilluminate.
        b) Some invade tissue planes around
           the oesophagus and trachea and
           may cause respiratory obstruc-
           tion. Sometimes, haemorrhage
           occurs into the cyst, resulting
           in a rapid increase in size;
           the patient becomes irritable,
           febrile and often with noisy
           breathing.

411.   a) Trauma.
        b) Malignant disease.

412.   Wilm's tumour, or nephroblastoma,
        presents usually in the first
        five years of life with an
        abdominal mass, lassitude and
        malaise. The worst cases have
        a five year survival of about
        50% and the most favourable
        100% survival.

413.   a) Reflux uropathy - vesicoureteric
           reflux.
        b) Obstructive uropathy - P.U.J.
           obstruction or less commonly,
           ureterovesical or urethral
           valves.
        c) Renal stones.
        d) Anatomical variants - many of
           these are clinically insignifi-
           cant, but duplex ureters with
           reflux, obstruction, uretero-
           celes and ectopic ureters are
           important.

Rectal Surgery

414. Briefly state the usual presenting
      symptoms of ulcerative colitis.

415. Where does the bowel distend most
      in large bowel obstruction, due
      to carcinoma for instance?

416. Which features of ulcerative colitis
      are particularly associated with
      the development of malignant
      change?

417. What observations should be recorded
      in the notes after performing
      sigmoidoscopy?

418. Classify haemorrhoids 1° - 3°.

419. Which types of piles are helped by
      injection sclerotherapy?

414.   Watery diarrhoea with mucus ± blood,
        and crampy abdominal pains.

415.   In the caecum. Thus caecal tenderness
        is an indication for urgent surgery
        to forestall perforation and
        general peritonitis.

416.   Onset of disease in youth.
        Clinically severe first attack.
        Involvement of the whole colon
            ('total colitis').
        Chronic continuous symptoms.
        Long duration of disease
            (i.e. over 10 years).
        Severe epithelial dysplasia.

417.   Luminal contents.
        Size of lumen (narrowing, ballooning).
        Mucosal appearances.
        Height achieved, difficulties
            encountered, response of patient.

418. 1^0 - piles bleed only.
        2^0 - piles bleed and come down with
                defaecation, but reduce
                spontaneously.
        3^0 - piles permanently prolapsed.

419.   Piles which bleed and prolapse only a
        little are suitable for injections.
        Those that prolapse considerably
        (especially 3^0 piles) are unsuit-
        able.

420. What do you think of a diagnosis of
      'painful piles' of a month's
      duration?

421. How should you investigate a patient
      who reports painless rectal
      bleeding without change in bowel
      habit?

422. In which order should you perform
      barium enema, digital rectal
      examination and sigmoidoscopy?

420.   This is almost certainly not piles
        but an anal fissure.
        Piles may cause some local discomfort,
        itching and a feeling of something
        coming down, but they are not
        painful unless acutely thrombosed
        (rare).
        Anal fissure gives sustained severe
        pain at each defaecation lasting
        for several hours.
        Diagnosis is made by inspection on
        parting nates. Digital examination
        is cruel and unnecessary.
        Treatment is urgent admission and anal
        stretch under G.A., or else passage
        of an anal dilator lubricated with
        anaesthetic jelly b.d. for a fort-
        night. If this fails, surgery is
        required. When the fissure has
        healed, full sigmoidoscopy must be
        performed to exclude pathology
        higher up.

421.   The minimum is full history and
        examination with digital rectal
        examination, sigmoidoscopy to at
        least 15 cm and a blood count.
        If piles are found, treat these.
        Whether all these cases require
        barium enema is controversial.
        If no cause can be found, barium
        enema must be performed.

422.   Digital examination first (never
        push an instrument where you
        have not felt and cannot see).
        Sigmoidoscopy) If you do the enema
        Barium enema) first the barium will
) coat the rectal wall
) and you will have to
) wait for several days
) before you are able to
) obtain adequate views
) through a sigmoidoscope.

423.   Why is a normal barium enema alone
        insufficient to exclude a large
        bowel cancer?

424.   Is rectal biopsy at sigmoidoscopy
        risk free?

425.   What are the classic sigmoidoscopic
        findings in a patient with acute
        ulcerative colitis?

423.   This examination is excellent for
        larger lesions in smaller tubes
        (e.g. colon) where it will demon-
        strate irregularities and
        narrowings, but is less good for
        cavities (e.g. rectum).
        Unless a small rectal cancer is
        caught in profile by the barium
        enema it will be missed in face-on
        views. Double contrast enema
        improves the accuracy considerably
        to 95% of polyps and carcinoma of
        1 cm. or larger diameter.
        Sigmoidoscopy is essential to exclude
        a rectal cancer.
        Digital rectal examination is needed
        to exclude an anal canal cancer.
        Only colonoscopy, which is unpleasant,
        expensive, time consuming and
        difficult will detect tiny colonic
        neoplasms.

424.   Not entirely.
        Below the pelvic reflection of the
        peritoneum (i.e. below 12 cm from
        the anus) biopsy is safe.
        Above this it is possible (rarely) to
        perforate the rectal wall.
        Very high up (25 cm) in the sigmoid
        colon, biopsy is more hazardous.
        Severe bleeding is rarely a problem
        with these sigmoidoscopic biopsies.

425.   Diffusely red velvety oedematous mucosa
        which bleeds on contact.
        There may be luminal mucus and blood.
        Biopsy at 12 cm is quite safe and
        may be very helpful.

426.   Is acute diverticulitis a common
        cause of emergency surgical
        admission in the elderly?
        What is the differential diagnosis?

427.   How would you manage a man of 68
        years admitted with acute
        diverticulitis?

428.   What five symptoms are typical of
        colonic carcinoma?

426.   Yes. It presents as left iliac fossa
        pain and tenderness with pyrexia
        in an older person with a history
        of constipation.
        Differential diagnosis:
        1) Carcinoma of descending colon
           + partial obstruction.
        2) Mesenteric ischaemia.
        3) Ovarian pathology.
        4) Other.

427.   The full-blown picture may need
           iv fluid and nasogastric
           suction, analgesics and anti-
           biotics with careful observation
           to identify developing peritonitis
           which requires operation.
        Mild cases just need a course of
           antibiotics and later high residue
           diet.
        Most cases fall between these two.
        Always remember the diagnosis is one
           of exclusion, and may be wrong.
        When recovered, the patient needs a
           sigmoidoscopy and an out-patient
           barium enema.

428.   Change in bowel habit.
        Passage of blood, slime mixed up
           with the stool.
        Abdominal pain.
        Abdominal mass.
        Increasing weakness ± weight loss.

429.   How common is diverticular disease?
        Does its distribution differ geograph-
            ically?
        How is it managed?

430.   What is the usual surgical treatment
        for acute or chronic ulcerative
        colitis?

429.   In western countries, diverticular
       disease is very common and is
       said to affect half the population
       over 50.
       Diverticular disease is associated
       with 'civilised' ways of life, it
       is rare in the third world and is
       thought to be due to different
       eating habits.
       The vast majority of cases are
       asymptomatic, only coming to light
       as incidental findings, and require
       no treatment.
       The majority of symptomatic cases are
       managed conservatively with a high
       residue diet, bran, etc.
       Surgical excision (usually of sigmoid
       colon) is used for:
       1) Complications of the disease
          e.g. stricture, perforation,
          bleeding, fistula.
       2) Severe symptoms.
       3) "Exclusion of a carcinoma" (with
          the introduction of colonoscopy
          this is becoming an increasingly
          rare indication).

430.   <u>Acute</u>: severe acute ulcerative colitis
       may develop into toxic dilatation of
       the colon, perforation and death.
       The key observations are abdominal
       distension, some tenderness,
       dilatation +++ of colon on plain
       x-ray.
       The safest operation is emergency
       colectomy + ileostomy alone. The
       rectal stump is oversewn and removed
       at a later date or, in suitable cases,
       an ileo-rectal anastomosis is
       constructed
       <u>Chronic</u>: surgery is performed either
       for intractable symptoms or because
       of the mounting cancer risk, which
       reaches 20% after 20 years colitis.
       Abdomino-perineal excision of the
       rectum + colon with ileostomy or
       preservation of the rectum with
       ileo-rectal anastomosis in suitable
       cases.

431.   What positive things does the
       operation of panproctocolectomy
       offer a patient with ulcerative
       colitis?

432.   Would you rather have bad Crohn's
       disease or severe ulcerative
       colitis?

431.   1) They will <u>feel</u> well. Most
           ulcerative colitics will tell
           you that they never compre-
           hended how generally ill they
           felt until after their colon
           had been removed, and they
           became well again.
        2) Loss of all their colonic symptoms.
        3) Complete protection from colonic
           carcinoma.
        4) Protection from the extra colonic
           complaints of U.C., e.g. arthro-
           pathy, and some hope that, if
           they already have this, it may
           regress.
        5) Continuation of a reasonable sex
           life (impotence after this
           operation is rare in good centres).

432.   Severe ulcerative colitis. Because
        once the decision has been taken
        to have a proctocolectomy and an
        ileostomy is accepted, you can
        look forward to the operation
        achieving complete cure with a
        return to normal life.
        Crohn's disease can be a terrible
        affliction in some patients
        involving multiple operations,
        fistulae etc. with chronic
        intractable ill-health, disrupting
        both physical and mental well
        being.

433.   Compare and contrast the typical
        features of ulcerative colitis
        and Crohn's disease.

434.   Compare and contrast the typical
        presentations of carcinoma of the
        descending and ascending colon.

433. Surgical interest tends to concen-
      trate on those cases with
      features of both diseases, and
      students may get the impression
      that the whole subject is blurred.
      This is not so. There are two
      different disease patterns and
      the majority of patients fall
      quite definitely into one or the
      other.
      Ulcerative colitis
          presents as bloody diarrhoea+++++
          affects the colon starting at the
            rectum
          does not affect the small bowel
            except rarely the terminal ileum
          does have a malignancy risk
          cured by panproctocolectomy with
            ileostomy
          histology - mucosal disease
      Crohn's disease
          presents as episodes of obstruction
            with slight bloody diarrhoea
          affects small bowel with skip
            lesions
          affects large bowel in only 20%
          tends to keep recurring with
            complications
          not pre-malignant, or minimal
            risk
          operations only treat the current
            episode and are often not curative
          histology - affects all coats of the
            bowel

434. Ascending colon
          wide tube with fluid faeces, hence
            presents late.
          presents as anaemia or mass.

      Descending colon
          narrow tube, solid faeces -
            obstructs early before any mass
            palpable.
          presents as obstruction or rectal
            bleeding/change in bowel habit.

435.   What determines whether a patient
        with rectal carcinoma has an
        anterior resection retaining the
        anus, or an abdomino-perineal
        excision + a permanent colostomy?

436.   How do you assess the prognosis for
        a patient who has recently under-
        gone left hemicolectomy for
        carcinoma of the colon?

435.   The site and size of the tumour.
        a) You can feel 10 cm inside
              at P.R.
           If you cannot touch the cancer,
              there is room to anastomose
              below and anterior resection
              is done.
           6-10 cm - practice differs.
           Below 6 cm - most surgeons will
              do an abdomino-perineal resection
              and permanent colostomy.
              Colo-anal procedures are still
              experimental.
        b) If the tumour is very large, or
              fixed, reconstruction after
              excision may prove impossible.
        c) If the tumour is poorly differ-
              entiated a more radical excision
              is usual and this usually means
              abdomino-perineal operation.

436.   Assuming that the patient is otherwise
        fit, prognosis depends on the histo-
        logical stage of the tumour.
        a) Dukes Grades:
           A - confined to bowel wall - 5 yr.
                survival. 80%
           B - wall breached, local spread,
                nodes negative. 5 yr. survival.
                70%
           C_1- B + local node involvement.
                5 yr. survival. 60%
           C_2- B + distant node involvement.
                5 yr. survival. 30%
           D - C + distant metastases. 5 yr.
                survival. 2-3%
        b) Cellular histology
              - well differentiated with
                lymphatic response is better
                than anaplastic.
              - carcinoid tumours(rare) carry
                a particularly good prognosis.

437.   How do you distinguish a peri-
       anal abscess from an infected
       pilonidal sinus? Does this
       distinction matter?

438.   Describe the immediate management
       of a patient who presents with
       as established peri-anal
       abscess.

439.   How should peri-anal abscess
       patients be followed up at
       O.P.D.?

437.   Distinguish them by position.
        Abscesses lying level with or
            anterior to the anus are obvi-
            ously peri-anal.
        Inflamed lumps lying behind the
            anus are more difficult. In
            fact this is quite an unusual
            place for a peri-anal abscess.
            An infected pilonidal sinus lies
            much higher up in the midline in
            the natal cleft, superficial to
            the sacrum. It is usually a long
            way from the anus. Look for the
            midline pit.
        Distinction is useful. Peri-anal
            abscess requires immediate formal
            incision and drainage under G.A.
        An infected pilonidal sinus may
            initially be managed by antibiotics
            or a quick incision in casualty,
            with later definitive surgery in
            the quiescent phase.

438.   Take a full history and examination,
            except that digital rectal exami-
            nation is cruel and unnecessary.
            Confine yourself to careful inspec-
            tion of the area.
        Immediate E.U.A. Perform digital
            rectal examination and sigmoid-
            oscopy under G.A.
            Incise and drain the abscess.
        Take some of its wall for histology.
        Send several mls. of pus for bacteri-
            ological culture including Tb.

439.   See them initially to ensure that the
            incised abscess heals soundly.
        Check that adequate sigmoidoscopy was
            done at the operation.
        See them once more at 1 year to check
            that there has been no recurrence.
            Late recurrence suggests some
            underlying anal fistula.

440.   Outline your post-operative management
        of a haemorrhoidectomy patient.

441.   What two major complications may
        occur after haemorrhoidectomy?
        How should they be managed?

440.   Immediate - adequate analgesia -
           e.g. Papaveretum 15 mg i.m.
           3-4 hourly p.r.n.
        Antiemetics - e.g. Perphenazine
           5 mg i.m. 4 hourly p.r.n.

        Start aperients e.g. Milpar 10 ml
           b.d. orally.
        Daily or b.d. soothing baths.
        First week - aperients to secure
           a bowel action within 6 days.
        At discharge - gentle rectal examin-
           ation, if normal   O.P.D. 1/12.
        If tight ⟶ anal dilator daily
           O.P.D. 1/52.

441.   a) 2^0 haemorrhage - rare 7th-10th
              day. May be profuse.
              Needs readmission + trans-
              fusion + re-operation.
        b) Anal stenosis - disastrous
              consequence of leaving
              inadequate 'skin bridges'.
              A 'tight' anus should be
              noted at p.r. before
              discharge.
              Such patients must never
              be left a month before
              O.P.D.
              Start anal dilatation(dilator
              passed b.d. by patient or
              District Nurse)
              See weekly at O.P.D.
              May need re-admissions for
              anal dilatation under G.A.
              until healed.
              Established gross post-
              haemorrhoidectomy anal
              stenosis is very difficult
              to cure.

Transplantation Surgery

442.　Which living tissues or organs may
　　　be successfully transplanted
　　　from a donor to a recipient
　　　patient (homograft)?

443.　Which tissues or organs may be
　　　successfully freely transplanted
　　　from one part of a patient to
　　　another (autograft)?

444.　Give approximate figures for the
　　　one year survival rate after
　　　a first renal transplantation
　　　of
　　a) the transplanted kidney
　　b) the patient
　　Why are these figures not identical?

445.　Why does a transplantation programme
　　　for kidneys involve fewer
　　　recipient deaths than those for
　　　liver or heart transplants?

442. Blood; bone marrow; kidney; cornea; liver; heart; pancreas (experimental).

443. Skin; bone; cartilage; nerve; artery; vein; fascia; fat; parathyroid; pancreatic islets (experimental).

444. a) 60% (reported results range from 20-80%).
b) 90%.
(b) is greater than (a) because although a rejected kidney may die, most of the recipients can be returned to haemodialysis and consequently survive.

445. Because renal transplant patients can be provided with the safety net of haemodialysis. This can be used both pre-operatively to correct metabolic disorder and as auxiliary support during the immediate post-operative period and also during oliguric rejection episodes, as well as being the ultimate salvation should the graft fail.
There is no adequate artificial heart or liver available at present, so if these grafts do not function fully immediately or fail during rejection, the patient dies.

446.   Transplantation results can only be
         as good as the donor organs
         allow.
         Donor organs removed from "heart
         beating cadavers" are much to be
         preferred.
         Removal of these donor organs pre-
         supposes certification of "brain
         death". "Brain death" certifi-
         cation was clarified in a joint
         statement from the Defence Unions
         and the British Transplantation
         Society *(B.M.J. 1976 (ii) 1187-
         1188)*.
         Outline the main points of procedure.

446.   1) Brain death to be certified by
          two doctors professionally
          <u>independent</u> of the transplant
          team.
          One should be a consultant who is
          in charge of the donor case, or
          in his absence, his deputy who
          should have been registered for
          5+ years and who should have had
          adequate previous experience in
          the care of such cases; plus one
          other doctor.
       2) The patient must be off all
          depressants and toxic drugs
          (including anaesthetics,
          paralysing agents, tranquillisers
          etc.) for an accepted period of
          time.
       3) Metabolic derangement (e.g. uraemia)
          must have been corrected as far
          as possible.
       4) Normal blood sugar.
       5) Absent brain stem reflexes
          including: pupil reflexes (fixed,
          dilated pupils): pain sensation,
          gag reflex: caloric reflex.
       6) When the ventilation is stopped,
          blood gases must be shown to
          alter ($\uparrow pCO_2$, $\downarrow pO_2$) to levels
          that would cause gross respira-
          tory stimulation and yet no
          spontaneous respiratory effort
          is made.
       A special form is available for
          completion which covers all these
          points.

447.   Once 'brain death' has been certified
        in the approved manner, are the
        transplant team free to use the
        donor organs?

448.   Everyone agrees that there is a
        lamentable shortage of good
        quality donor kidneys.
        How do you think that the H.S. should
        respond if a staff nurse on an
        I.T.U. were to suggest that he
        might gently ask the relatives of
        a bad head injury whether they
        would view favourably the ultimate
        possibility of his organs being
        used for transplantations?

447.   Not always. In non-violent cases,
       provided that the patient has
       also been certified as dead and
       the relatives agree, the organs
       may be used, otherwise the body
       is under the jurisdiction of H.M.
       Coroner. His permission must be
       obtained as well as that of any
       relatives. He is most unlikely
       to overrule any objections from
       them.

448.   Our joint view is that we cannot
       envisage any circumstances in
       which it would be appropriate for
       the H.S. to make an unauthorised
       approach of this kind to relatives.
   The decision even to sound out the
       relatives is a grave and heavy one
       and should be reserved for the
       consultant in charge of the patient
       or, only in his absence, his
       immediate deputy.
   The correct response is for the H.S.
       to ask the I.T.U. sister whether
       she shares her staff nurse's
       opinion and then for him to report
       the sister's view to his seniors,
       for them to decide in consultation
       with the I.T.U. anaesthetists,
       transplant team and nursing staff
       what, if anything, should be done.
   One of the cruellest blows possible
       for the relatives of a dying young
       person is to have some well meaning
       but inexperienced doctor set in
       motion the wheels of "transplantation"
       only for the transplant surgeon
       eventually to reject the organ as
       technically unsuitable.

Urology

449. How far do you think the H.S's.
responsibility extends in the
operating theatre in identifying
the side for a nephrectomy?

450. Why is it important to distinguish
between acute painful retention
of urine and chronic painless
retention?

449.   It is the H.S's. job to ensure that
the actual I.V.P. films are
present, to have obtained the
patient's written consent for,
and marked the correct side.
(This is all delegated work.)
The responsibility for operating on
the correct side rests entirely
with the surgeon performing the
operation, and not on his assistants;
but a good H.S. will stop his chief
from operating on the wrong side!

450.   Because treatment is different.
Acute painful retention requires
immediate full decompression by
catheter.
Painless retention requires more
thought. Provided the sensory
pathways are intact, the condition
indicates a chronic status quo
without urgency. Decompression
(which is not always necessary)
should be part of an elective
planned therapeutic procedure as
rapid decompression of a chronically distended bladder may be
dangerous. Not only may it precip-
itate haemorrhage into the urinary
tract but also, if there is
co-existent uraemia, there may be
a profound resultant diuresis. If
the fluid and electrolyte losses
are not carefully replaced by
intravenous infusion, then death
may result.

451.   What are the main indications for
       prostatectomy?

452.   Define varicocele.
       Is this often an important diagnosis
       to make?

453.   What are the symptoms and signs of
       a ruptured urethra?
       What should a keen H.S. do about
       one?

451.   Prostatectomy is performed to relieve
            symptoms, diagnosis can be
            achieved by simple biopsy.
        - attacks of acute painful retention
            of urine.
        - troublesome chronic retention with
            overflow.
        - uraemia due to outflow obstruction.
        - symptoms of poor stream and
            disabling frequency*.
        - recurrent or persistent) in associ-
            urinary infection.   ) ation with
        - bladder stones.   ) prostatic
) obstruction

        *Frequency alone is not an indication
            for prostatectomy. These patients
            require urodynamic pressure studies,
            as prostatectomy in the wrong case
            can make the frequency worse.

452.   Varicosity of the cremasteric and
            pampiniform venous plexuses.
        Only in male infertility (treating
            a varicocele makes the testicle
            cooler and improves the sperm
            count) and very rarely a left
            varicocele may indicate a left
            hypernephroma (renal cell
            carcinoma).
        A large varicocele may also cause a
            dragging sensation in the scrotum.

453.   Pain, perineal haematoma, blood at
            the external meatus (remember to
            retract the foreskin and look!),
            urinary retention.
        The keen H.S. should refrain from
            doing anything himself.
        Inexpert instrumentation can convert
            a partial into a complete urethral
            tear. He should inform his
            superiors.

454.   What may mimic a renal calculus on
        a plain x-ray?

455.   Name some of the problems associated
        with Stilboestrol therapy for
        prostatic carcinoma?

456.   Outline your management of a painless
        unilateral testicular swelling.

457.   You see a boy of eleven in your
        evening surgery with slight
        dysuria and a painful, enlarged
        testicle. He tells you that he
        was kicked that afternoon at
        football, but it was not very
        bad. What should you do?

454.   Calcified lymph node.   Chip fractured
        Gallstone.   vertebra.
        Ingested pill.   Calcified adrenal.
        Phlebolith.   Calcified old
        Ossified tip of R12.   renal Tb.
        Calcified splenic   Artefact
           artery aneurysm.   (e.g. pyjama
                                   button).

455.   Fluid retention precipitating heart
            failure.
        Thrombo-embolism, D.V.T., P.E. etc.
        Embarrassing gynaecomastia.
        Impotence.
        Resistant cancer.

456.   The majority transilluminate, are
            cystic, being either hydroceles
            or epididymal cysts.
        Those that are solid testis should
            be explored through a groin
            incision, and are nearly always
            tumours. Never be tempted to
            try aspiration of a solid, enlarged
            testis. If it is malignant, you
            will encourage local seeding.

457.   Refer the boy to Casualty, nil by
            mouth, and personally contact
            a senior member of the duty surgical
            team.
        All testicular pain in young men and
            boys should be treated as <u>testicular
            torsion</u>.
        For practical purposes, urinary
            infection does not occur in this
            age group.
        Many boys get kicked during football -
            if there is a major haematoma it
            will benefit from decompression.
        This boy's testicle should be explored
            within the hour, looking for
            torsion.

458.   Once a suspected testicular torsion
       has been confirmed at operation
       and fixed, what else should be
       done?

459.   What are the principles underlying
       the management of young women
       with so-called recurrent 'cystitis'?

460.   If a normally asymptomatic sexually
       active young woman is prone to
       attacks of cystitis what simple
       advice can you give her on
       prophylaxis?

458.   The other side is also at risk and
        should be fixed. Most surgeons
        do this at the same operation.
    The underlying defect is a long
        mesotestis. Later, the testicles
        of male relatives should be
        examined with a view to prophy-
        lactic advice + surgery.

459.   Obtain a full urological and gynae-
        cological history from the patient;
        cystitis means different things to
        different women, and examine the
        external genitalia for obvious
        pathology.
    Do repeated M.S.U. cultures and vaginal
        swabs to establish whether the bouts
        of symptoms are associated with
        bacterial infection, and whether
        the quiescent phases are accompanied
        by sterile urine or asymptomatic
        bacteriuria.
    Do I.V.P. + micturating cystogram
        + cystoscopy to establish normal or
        abnormal anatomy.
    When you have all this information you
        are in a position to give logical
        local and systemic treatment.

460.   Avoid vaginal douches and antiseptics.
        The normal vaginal flora are the
        best cleansers available.
    Wear stockings and cotton knickers
        rather than tights.
    Drink plenty of fluid on a regular
        basis.
    Take regular baths, and also wash
        carefully before intercourse.
    When having intercourse indulge in
        sufficient foreplay to make both
        partners really moist, and insist
        on a careful, gentle slow initial
        penetration.
    Try to pass urine relatively soon
        after intercourse.
    This may be achieved by morning coitus
        before rising for the day.

461. What is a sterile pyuria?
      What is the commonest cause
        nowadays?

462. Once a patient has commenced anti-
        biotic treatment for a urinary
        infection, and their symptoms
        remit, should they "complete the
        course"?

463. Should all women with urinary tract
        infection undergo bacteriological
        screening?

461.   Sterile pyuria = W.B.C. ++
        Bacterially sterile urine.
        1. Bacterial urinary infection
           partly treated by antibiotics -
           far the commonest cause.
        2. Recent urinary instrumentation
           (e.g. catheter removal).
        3. Urological Tb (the classical
           cause of this finding, but now
           quite rare).
        4. Some cases of urological calculi.

462.   Views on this topic are less unanimous
           than before, but it is still gener-
           ally accepted that a patient should
           complete a 10-14 day course of
           urinary antibiotics provided
        1. The initial M.S.U. result did grow
           bacteria.
        2. The bacteria cultured were sensitive
           to the antibiotics.
        3. There is no other major contra-
           indication.

463.   In theory yes, in practice cost-
           effectiveness dictates no.
        In hospital practice, it probably
           remains cost-effective to test
           everyone.
        In general practice, all patients with
           recurrent infections must have
           adequate M.S.U. tests, before, during,
           at the end of and some time after
           antibiotic treatment. It is probably
           safe, if a little undesirable, to
           treat "first offenders" on an
           empirical basis without, or with only
           one, M.S.U.

464.   After how many proven episodes of
        bacteriologically positive
        urinary tract infections should
        you refer a little girl or boy
        for full urological investigation?

465.   How does the patient notice haemo-
        spermia?
        Is it important?

466.   How may carcinoma of the prostate
        present clinically?

464.   The length of the male urethra means
        that any proven urine infection
        in a boy is abnormal, and demands
        referral for investigation.
        The short female urethra makes girls
        more prone to cystitis. A second
        attack requires referral. It is
        very helpful for the specialist
        to have M.S.U. results from both
        episodes.

465.   Many men find this a most embarrassing
        and frightening complaint.
        It is usually noticed the next day by
        the female partner clearing up a
        used condom containing blood-
        stained semen. Sometimes sheets
        may be stained, and occasionally
        she herself may report a blood-
        stained vaginal discharge to her
        doctor.
        The man should be examined and an
        M.S.U. taken, but haemospermia
        almost never has any sinister
        significance. There is no treat-
        ment and it disappears.

466.   Typically it presents as a rapid onset
        of bladder outflow obstruction
        ("prostatism") ± slight terminal
        painless haematuria.
        Rarely bony secondaries may be the
        presenting feature.
        Diagnosis is by rectal palpation of a
        hard and irregular prostate
        confirmed by biopsy.
        A raised acid phosphatase level may
        indicate extraprostatic spread.
        Histological confirmation should be
        obtained before any treatment is
        commenced.

467.   What principles govern the treatment
        of prostatic carcinoma?

467. Controversial.
      Stilboestrol is the mainstay of
         treatment and improves the quality
         of life but does not lengthen it.
      a) Focus of carcinoma in a resected
            benign gland: No treatment.
      b) Resected malignant growth, no local
            metastasis, asymptomatic: No
            treatment.
      c) Bony secondaries -) Treatment contro-
            asymptomatic   ) versial -
      d) Asymptomatic extra-) probably
            prostatic spread) Stilboestrol or
            on P.R.   ) castration
      e) Pain from bony)Stilboestrol
            secondaries,)treatment $\pm$ radio-
            prostatism   )therapy or castra-
            symptoms   )tion or pituitary
                         ablation.

468.   Describe the technique of catheter-
       ization of a man with acute
       retention of urine.

468. Attempt to discover why he has retention and if you can foresee difficulties (previous stricture, difficult catheterization etc.) consult your registrar.

Assuming all is well, ensure your trolley has all you require.

Give a small dose of Pethidine iv before you begin.

Wash your hands, take one swab to wipe the glans, and squeeze in 2/3 of the tube of lignocaine jelly. Still holding the nozzle in the meatus, massage the gel up the urethra as far as the bulb with about five firm strokes of your hand. If you have done this properly, when you remove the nozzle, the gel should largely remain in the urethra and not pour out.

Now scrub fully, lay out your trolley, and place catheter, disinfectant, remaining lubricant and syringe of water in a kidney dish.

Start with a size 16F Foley catheter dipped in the gel.

Pull the penis taught vertically pointing at the ceiling.

Pass the catheter to the 'S' bend of the bulb.

Still pulling, point the penis at his feet and advance the catheter around the bulb and up into the bladder.

Inflate the balloon and connect the bag.

Offer to clear up the trolley if you hope to remain friends with your nursing staff.

469.   What should the H.S. do when he is
        having difficulty passing a
        catheter on a man?

470.   In some units disposable suprapubic
        stab-catheters (supracath) are
        used for treating acute urinary
        retention. What simple rules
        must be followed if insertion is
        to be safe?

469.   The golden rule is to give up early
        before you have done any damage.
        Make sure that the patient has
           received sedation and analgesia
           (e.g. Pethidine, Chlorpromazine).
        Withdraw the catheter completely and
           look at its tip.
        As soon as you start to make the
           urethra bleed, you must stop and
           call someone more senior.
        Try a second time, pulling the penis
           up and down even more firmly, but
           still inserting the catheter
           gently.
        Try gently once more with a smaller
           catheter (e.g. size 12F).
        NEVER USE FORCE
        You are not permitted to use an
           introducer. The inexpert can do
           real damage with this instrument.
           You need your Registrar.

470.   The lower abdomen should be free from
           scars.
        The bladder must be obviously palpable
           or percussible above the symphysis
           pubis.
        A little intravenous sedation and
           analgesia is helpful.
        After inserting the local anaesthetic,
           always perform a trial needle
           aspiration of the bladder at the
           proposed puncture site. Unless
           clear urine is obtained you must not
           proceed. Large cannulae have been
           thrust into aortic aneurysms!
        When the catheter is safely in, inflate
           its balloon *before* allowing the
           urine to drain and the bladder to
           collapse.
        If you become unsure about what you
           are doing, stop and ask.

471.   How would you investigate a single
       episode of painless haematuria?

472.   What is a Wilm's tumour?

473.   How does renal adenocarcinoma usually
       present?
       Correctly treated, does this condition
       usually carry a good or bad
       prognosis?

471.   All cases of <u>painless</u> haematuria
         must be regarded as urological
         cancer until proved otherwise.
         All cases require a minimum of:
         history and examination
         M.S.U.
         blood count
         urea
         I.V.U.
         cystourethroscopy
         The vast majority will have small
            bladder cancer(s).
         Some will have upper renal tract
            cancers.
         In about 20% no cause will be found,
            and the bleeding ascribed to
            "prostatic veins" etc. Urinary
            cytology looking for malignant
            cells may be helpful in this
            group which should be carefully
            followed up in O.P.D. in case a
            small tumour has been missed.

472.   An embryonal tumour affecting infants'
            and children's kidneys.
         It usually presents as an abdominal
            mass ± haematuria.
         If treated at an 'early stage',it
            carries a relatively favourable
            prognosis.
         This tumour should be treated in a
            centre specialising in paediatric
            urology.
         Combined therapy means that the
            tumour carries a fairly favourable
            prognosis.

473.   Haematuria ± loin mass, ± pain.
         In the usual case where the tumour
            is confined to the kidney which
            is removed en bloc as 'radical
            nephrectomy', the long term
            prognosis is quite good, in most
            large series 50% survival at 5 years.

474. Do the majority of patients presenting
      with ureteric colic due to a stone
      require surgery to remove it?

475. How do you distinguish at the bedside
      between a patient with a right
      ureteric colic and acute appendi-
      citis?

476. How do you treat acute ureteric colic?

477. Is there any point referring a boy
      with hypospadias to a specialist
      until he is 3 years old, and the
      organ large enough for an
      operation?

474.   No.
       The vast majority of ureteric stones
          are passed spontaneously, particu-
          larly if less than 6 mm in their
          smallest diameter.

475.   Ureteric colic:
          Apyrexial, restless patient rolling
          about trying to get comfortable.
          Abdomen remains soft and not tender.
          Urine positive to blood (usually).
       Appendicitis:
          Slight pyrexia, patient lies still,
          movement hurts.
          Tenderness and guarding in the R.I.F.
          Urine clear (usually but not always).

476.   1. Analgesia - Pethidine, initially
             low dose i.v. while you sort out
             the diagnosis.
       2. Diagnosis - history, examination,
             test urine, plain x-ray,
             emergency I.V.U.
       3. I.V.U. - normal - change diagnosis.
          I.V.U. - (partial blockage +
                   (normal other side -
                    treat conservatively
          I.V.U. - (partial blockage +
                   (absent other side -
                    treat actively if
                    obstruction persists.
          I.V.U. - complete blockage
                   further tests, e.g.
                   renogram.

477.   Yes. Such boys should be referred as
          soon as the condition is diagnosed.
       To assess the problem technically,
          i.e. whether one or two stage
          repair.
       To explain the condition to the parents
          and outline the surgery required.
       To look for other associated conditions
          e.g. meatal stenosis, undescended
          testis, or rarities which may need
          correction sooner.

478.   Pre-operative urine culture is an
        important part of the management
        of patients about to undergo
        prostatectomy. Why?

479.   What is a paraphimosis?
        Is there any urgency about it?
        How would you reduce one?

480.   How should you treat a boy of 8 years
        who has caught his penis in his
        trouser zip?

478.   If the urine is known to be infected
        it is wise to start appropriate
        antibiotic treatment just prior
        to surgery and continue it until
        after removal of the catheter.
        If the urine is sterile, antibiotics
        can be reserved for treatment when
        and if infection occurs rather than
        employ routine prophylaxis which is
        more likely to encourage antibiotic
        resistant organisms, and to affect
        morbidity.

479.   When the foreskin is tight, forceful
        retraction may just coax its edge
        beyond the glans which pops out in
        full protraction with the tight
        neck clasping its corona. This
        constriction causes swelling of
        the foreskin and glans which
        rapidly becomes vast and oedematous.
        This is a paraphimosis.
        Treatment is urgent because it hurts
        and if not reduced may lead to
        necrosis!
        If seen early, sedate the patient,
        cover the penis with KY jelly and
        attempt forceful manual reduction.
        If this fails, administer a G.A.
        and cut the constricting band, and
        then either convert this to a
        dorsal slit of the foreskin or
        circumcise.
        In children the mental effect of an
        attempted manual reduction may be
        great, so always use a G.A.

480.   You may be certain that he and his
        family will have attempted forceful
        removal before bringing him to
        Casualty - there is no need for you
        to try too, because of the physical
        pain and mental trauma that this
        will cause. Arrange for a G.A. and
        then inspect and correct the damage.

Index

ABDOMEN 1-9, 37, 39, 40-44, 46, 48-58, 64, 66,
         67, 70, 71, 76-80, 83-92, 95-118, 131,
         132, 180, 186, 192-195, 201, 203,
         273-276, 279, 359, 375-379, 393-396,
         400, 402-406, 411, 413-417, 421,
         423-436, 470.
ABSCESS Amoebic 71.
         Breast 12, 21, 189.
         Cerebral 306.
         General 119.
         Ischio-rectal 183.
         Pelvic 194, 195.
         Perianal 437, 438, 439.
         Subphrenic 192, 193.
ACHALASIA 10, 215.
ACIDITY TESTS 111.
ACIDOSIS 147.
ACUTE ABDOMEN 1, 2, 4, 5. (See Appendicitis)
ADHESIONS 85, 86.
ALKALOSIS 92.
AMPUTATION 184.
ANAEMIA 76, 97, 109.
ANAESTHESIA 78, 121, 136-145, 212.
ANEURYSM 171, 174, 180.
ANKLE 349, 363.
ANTERIOR COMPARTMENT SYNDROME 170.
ANTIBIOTICS See Infection/Therapeutics/Bacteri-
                   ology.
APPENDICITIS 2, 3, 8, 9, 273, 278, 401, 475.
ARTERIAL SURGERY 163-181.
ARTHRITIS 362, 366, 373.
ASCITES 37.
BACTERIOLOGY 36, 182-201.
BEDSORES 35, 36.
BILE DUCTS 70, 78, 80, 106.
BILIRUBIN 77.
BLADDER 149, 450, 459, 460.
BLEEDING See Haemorrhage.
BLOOD 62, 66, 76, 78, 105, 173, 202, 283-287.
BRAIN DEATH 446-448.

BREAST Abscess 12, 189.
        Aspiration of cyst 20.
        Carcinoma 14, 25, 32.
        Duct ectasia 23.
        Dysplasia 15, 16.
        Endocrine manipulation 31.
        Fibroadenoma 13.
        Intraduct papilloma 27.
        Lump 18, 19, 24.
        Mammograms 28.
        Mastectomy 29. 30.
        Mastitis 23.
        Nipple 21, 22, 26.
        Nipple discharge 23.
        Screening 116.
BRONCHUS 69.
BURN 135.
CALCANEUS 345.
CARCINOID 72.
CARDIOTHORACIC 126, 176, 177, 202-228.
CATARACT 340.
CATHETERS 152, 468-470.
CHEMOTHERAPY 31, 81, 472.
CHOLECYSTITIS 40, 41, 42, 79, 186, 226.
CHORIONCARCINOMA 81.
CIMETIDINE 100.
CLAUDICATION 165, 167, 168, 181.
COLON Barium studies 182, 423.
        Carcinoma 33, 426, 428, 434, 435.
        Diverticulitis 426, 427.
        Ulcerative colitis 414, 416, 425, 430-433.
CONSTIPATION 89.
CROHN's 1, 432, 433.
CROSS-MATCHING 66.
CUSHING's 245, 246.
CYST Breast 16, 20.
        Dermoid 249, 408.
        Hydatid 71.
        Hygroma 74, 410.
        Neck 241, 409, 410.
        Ovary 1, 274, 276.
        Sebaceous 120, 249.
        Thyroglossal 241.
CYTOLOGY 20, 37, 223.
DEAFNESS 267, 268, 271.
DEBRIDEMENT 113.
DEEP VEIN THROMBOSIS 82, 224, 225, 374.
DIARRHOEA 109, 194, 201, 237, 247, 414.
DIVERTICULITIS 426, 427, 429.
DUMPING SYNDROME 106, 107.

DUODENUM   Atresia 393.
            Ulcer 64, 67, 101, 102, 104, 105, 115.
DRAINS   Intercostal 206, 210, 211, 222.
           Time of removal 45.
           T-tube 46, 151.
DRIPS   See Intravenous Infusion.
DYSPEPSIA 56.   See Duodenal and Gastric Ulcer.
DYSPHAGIA 56, 216.
DYSURIA 3, 457.
EAR NOSE THROAT 231, 248-271, 315.
ECTOPIC PREGNANCY 1, 272, 280.
ECZEMA (of nipple) 26.
ELECTROLYTES 92, 235.
EMBOLISM 166, 224, 225, 227, 228, 277.
ENDOCRINE SURGERY 229-247.
ENDOMETRIOSIS 1.
ENDOSCOPY 57, 99, 108, 124, 218.
EPIGLOTTIS 253.
EYE SURGERY 237, 258, 319, 326-343, 408.
EXOMPHALOS 378.
FEMUR 347, 350, 361, 365, 367, 372.
FISTULA 241.
FLUID BALANCE 146-162.
FRACTURE 309, 310, 314, 315, 344, 345, 352, 353,
            357, 359. 360, 361, 363, 365, 367, 368.
GALL STONES 39-44, 79, 118.
GANGRENE (of Bowel) 55.
GASTRIC ULCER 102.
GASTROENTERITIS 1.
GYNAECOLOGY 1, 3, 4, 18, 132, 195, 196, 237,
            272-280, 459, 460, 464, 465.
HAEMATEMESIS 64, 66, 97, 124.
HAEMATOLOGY See Blood 283-287.
HAEMOPTYSIS 207, 208.
HAEMORRHAGE 56, 60, 63, 64, 65, 67, 104, 105, 124,
            263, 264, 307, 313, 314, 338, 361,
            404, 405, 441, 453.
HAEMORRHOIDS 418, 419, 420, 440, 441.
HAMARTOMA 59.
HAND 354-356, 360, 362, 369, 370.
HEAD INJURY 188, 265, 307-312, 315-317.

HERNIA   Definition 47.
          Diaphragmatic 397.
          Epigastric 379.
          Femoral 48, 53,
          Hiatus 56, 57.
          Incisional 51.
          Inguinal 50, 58, 375, 376.
          Irreducible 49.
          Richter's 55.
          Strangulated 52.
          Umbilical 54.
          MISCELLANEOUS 85, 86, 377.
HIP JOINT 347, 350, 372, 373, 374.
HIRSCHSPRUNG's 395.
HUMERUS 360, 364.
HYDROCELE 384, 385.
HYPER/HYPOKALAEMIA 92, 147, 151, 155.
HYPOGLYCAEMIA 109, 247, 317.
HYPOSPADIAS, 382, 383, 477.
HYPOVOLAEMIA 92, 125, 126.
ILEUS 87, 88, 194, 394.
INCIDENCE 34.
INFECTION (See Abscess and Bacteriology also)
          Eye 326, 334.
          Face 258.
          Hand 356, 369, 370.
      .   Hospital 197.
          Lymphangitis 196.
          Perianal 438, 439.
          Pilonidal 437.
          Pyrexia in 82.
          Shock 126.
          Urine 461-464.
          Wound 200.
INTENSIVE CARE 68.
INTRA CRANIAL PRESSURE 318, 322.
INTRA VENOUS INFUSION 143-145, 148-161, 280, 427.
INTUSSUSCEPTION 85.
ISCHAEMIA 163, 164, 170, 175, 178, 179.
JAUNDICE 76-79.
KELLER's 348.
KIDNEY 1, 158, 240, 412, 442, 444, 445, 449, 454,
       472, 473.
KNEE JOINT 346.
LARYNX 213, 214, 231, 251, 252, 254-256.
LEIOMYOMA 99.
LIVER 70-72, 158, 192, 193.
LUNG 202, 204, 206-212, 222-225, 227, 228, 283.
LYMPHATIC 53, 196, 249, 261, 262.
LYMPHOMA 70, 72, 81, 99.

MALABSORPTION 109.
MALIGNANT TUMOURS   Bile Duct 80.
                     Bowel 85, 415, 423.
                     Breast 18, 20, 25, 29, 30-33.
                     Bronchus 69.
                     Chemotherapy for 81.
                     Children in 412.
                     Colon 33, 416.
                     Ear 271,
                     Kidney 412, 472, 473.
                     Liver 70.
                     Lung 204, 207.
                     Nasopharynx 261.
                     Occult 38, 72.
                     Oesophagus 203, 217, 218.
                     Pancreas 79, 247.
                     Parotid 93, 248-250.
                     Prostate 455, 466, 467.
                     Testis 387.
                     Thyroid 229, 239.
                     Tongue 259.
MECKEL's DIVERTICULUM 1, 404.
MECONIUM 394.
MELAENA 62, 66, 67, 97.
MESENTERIC ADENITIS 6.
MESENTERIC INFARCTION 83, 426.
MUSCLE POWER 130.
MYCOSIS FUNGOIDES 81.
NAEVUS 391.
NASO-GASTRIC TUBE 220, 221.
NECK LUMPS 17, 74, 75, 234, 239, 241, 249, 251,
          409, 410.
NERVE INJURY 323, 324.
NEUROMA 99.
NEUROSURGERY 306-325, 399, 446.
NURSING and ADMINISTRATION 8, 288-305, 449.
NUTRITION 129, 162.
OBESITY 128, 129.
OBSTRUCTION   Bile Duct 43, 80.
              Intestinal 85-89, 91, 92, 95, 104,
                138, 415.
              Laryngeal 213, 214, 243, 257.
              Urinary 466.
OEDEMA 207, 243, 258, 283.
OESOPHAGUS 10, 124, 203, 217-219, 392.
ORTHOPAEDICS 170, 344-374.
OVARY 1, 274, 276, 278, 426

PAEDIATRIC SURGERY 209, 214, 253, 301, 360, 372, 375-413.
PANCREAS 79, 80, 117, 118.
PARAPLEGIA 35, 320, 325.
PARATHYROID 240.
PAROTID 93, 94, 248, 250.
PATELLA 368.
PENIS 380-382, 479, 480.
PERFORATION 104, 115.
PLASTER CASTS 358, 359.
PROLAPSED DISC 323.
PROSTATE 199, 451, 455, 466, 467, 478.
PYREXIA 7, 82, 194, 283, 402, 403.
RADIOTHERAPY 205.
RAYNAUD 112.
RECTUM 395, 396, 404, 417, 420-425, 435, 437.
REIDEL's LOBE 71.
SALPINGITIS 1.
SCREENING 116, 398, 463.
SCROTUM 389, 390, 457.
SHOCK 125, 126, 159.
SICKLE CELL 142.
SIGMOIDOSCOPY 417, 424, 425, 439.
SKIN CANCER 122, 123.
SODIUM BALANCE 156.
SPLEEN 132, 133, 154, 287.
STEATORRHOEA 109.
STOMACH   Carcinoma 69, 97, 98, 99.
                    Dilatation Acute 84.
                    Drugs acting on 100.
                    Dumping 106, 107.
                    Endocrine 96.
                    Naso gastric tube 220, 221.
                    Post-gastrectomy symptoms 109, 201.
                    Pyloric stenosis 95, 406.
                    Surgery of 203.
                    Ulceration 102, 108.
STRANGULATION 90, 376.
SUTURES 134.
SYMPATHECTOMY 172, 342.
TESTIS 386-388, 456-458, 465.
TETANUS 190, 191.
THERAPEUTICS 14, 73, 90, 100, 121, 136, 157, 179, 183-187, 190, 191, 193, 195, 196, 198-201, 230, 250, 283, 316, 317, 326, 327, 330, 331, 336, 455, 462, 467.
THYROID 229-234, 236-239, 242-244.
TIBIA 367.
TONGUE 75, 251, 259.
TONSIL 260.

TRACHEOSTOMY 213, 214, 257.
TRANSPLANT SURGERY 442-448.
TRAUMA 113, 114, 211, 212, 266, 324, 328, 329,
        330, 332, 335-337, 341, 343-346, 350-355,
        357, 360, 361, 363-368, 371, 453, 457,
        480.   Also see Head Injury.
TROISIER's SIGN 69.
TUBERCULOSIS 207, 208, 259, 461.
ULCER   Duodenal 67, 101-103.
        Fissure 420.
        Gastric 103.
        Peptic 110, 111, 247.
        Skin 122.
ULTRASOUND 171, 179.
URETER 1, 474, 475, 476.
URETHRA 182, 453, 469.
URINE 152, 194. 403, 450, 461, 471, 478.
UROLOGY 413, 449-480.
VAGOTOMY 108, 111.
VARICOCOELE 452,
VARICOSE VEINS 137.
VIRCHOW NODE 69.
VOMITING 56, 66, 87, 89, 97, 106, 109, 138, 276,
         307, 318, 406.
WARTS 127.
WOUNDS 113, 131, 309.
WRIST 353, 357.
X-RAY 10, 28, 40, 41, 115, 133, 165, 167, 182,
       204, 209, 215, 217, 221, 222, 232, 274,
       309, 344, 351, 354, 357, 363, 368, 393,
       422, 423, 430, 454, 471.